Current Cardiovascular Therapy

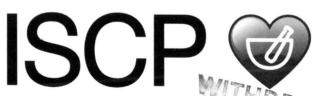

ISCP

International Society of Cardiovascular Pharmacotherapy

Albert Ferro • David A. Garcia
Editors

Antiplatelet and Anticoagulation Therapy

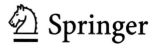

Springer

Editors
Albert Ferro
King's College London
London
UK

David A. Garcia
University of New Mexico
Albuquerque
New Mexico
USA

ISBN 978-1-4471-4296-6   ISBN 978-1-4471-4297-3 (eBook)
DOI 10.1007/978-1-4471-4297-3
Springer London Heidelberg New York Dordrecht

Library of Congress Control Number: 2012950008

Preface

Drugs used to prevent and treat thrombotic diseases are amongst the most widely used in clinical medicine. Aspirin, once used principally for its anti-inflammatory and analgesic actions, is now predominantly used as an anti-platelet agent. Despite the fact that it was one of the first drugs to come into common usage, having been developed by Felix Hoffmann in 1897 and subsequently marketed by Bayer, aspirin remains the most widely used drug in the world. Warfarin was originally developed and used as a rodenticide, and in 1954 was approved for medical use in humans; since then, warfarin and related coumarin derivatives have been the only orally active anticoagulant drugs available to the physician.

For decades, therefore, aspirin has dominated the anti-platelet landscape, and the vitamin K antagonists have done the same in the field of anticoagulation. These therapeutic areas have not remained entirely static. The thienopyridine drugs came along and gave added anti-platelet value when added to aspirin: first ticlopidine and its successor clopidogrel, which proved to be better tolerated and gave much less in the way of hematologic adverse effects. Advances also came in parenteral anticoagulants, with the development of low molecular-weight heparins, a significant advance in terms of both ease of administration and lack of need for close monitoring as compared with standard unfractionated heparin; the hirudins and, most recently, the synthetic pentasaccharides, each of which found its particular niche. But a major challenge has been to find an oral anticoagulant which is easier and more straightforward to use than warfarin.

These are all incremental advances which have taken place over the course of roughly two decades. However, the last five years have seen major advances in both anti-platelet and anticoagulant drugs, in each case with new agents becoming available which provide a step change from therapies previously well established. Newer more efficacious anti-platelet drugs have reached the marketplace: prasugrel, a third-generation thienopyridine, which is not only more efficacious than clopidogrel but is also more predictable in its pharmacodynamics; ditto ticagrelor, an entirely new class of anti-platelet drug but which, like the thienopyridines, inhibits the $P2Y_{12}$ receptor. As always, increased efficacy comes with a price, in particular increased bleeding risk. New oral anticoagulants are also now available for clinical use: the direct thrombin inhibitor dabigatran etexilate and the direct factor Xa inhibitors apixaban and rivaroxaban. They have simpler dosing regimes than the vitamin K antagonists and do not require routine monitoring of their anticoagulant effect. Again, however, there are trade-offs: none of these drugs has an antidote, and many patients with significant renal insufficiency will be unable to use these newer medicines.

This book is designed as an accessible, up-to-date reference for clinicians using anti-platelet and anti-coagulant drugs. Much use is made of pictures and figures to ease the assimilation of information. It covers the nature and pharmacology of these drugs, and also how they should be used in specific clinical situations. A chapter is also included on the contentious topic of anti-platelet monitoring. All of the chapters are written by authors who are established authorities in their fields as well as experienced educators and exponents of their subjects. The result is a unique book which is not only comprehensive but also easy-to-read and useful for the busy clinician.

Albert Ferro
USA   David Garcia

Contents

Contributors

Jack Ansell, M.D. Department of Medicine,
Lenox Hill Hospital, New York, NY, USA

Adrian J.B. Brady, M.D., FRCP, FESC, FAHA Department
of Medical Cardiology, University of Glasgow, Glasgow, UK

Nathan P. Clark, Pharm.D., BCPS., CACP
Department of Pharmacy, Clinical Pharmacy
Anticoagulation & Anemia Service,
Kaiser Permanente Colorado, Aurora, CO, USA

Jesse Dawson, M.D., B.Sc., (Hons), MBChB (Hons), FRCP
Institute of Cardiovascular and Medical Sciences,
College of Medicine, Veterinary & Life Sciences,
Western Infirmary, Glasgow, UK

Christopher Dittus, DO, MPH Department of Medicine,
Lenox Hill Hospital, New York, NY, USA

Albert Ferro Department of Clinical Pharmacology,
School of Medicine (Cardiovascular Division),
King's College London, London, UK

David Garcia Department of Internal Medicine,
University of New Mexico, Albuquerque, USA

Paul A. Gurbel, M.D. Sinai Center for Thrombosis
Research, Sinai Hospital of Baltimore, Baltimore, MD, USA

Johns Hopkins University School of Medicine,
Baltimore, MD, USA

Stan Heptinstall B.Sc., Ph.D. Division of Cardiovascular
Medicine, School of Clinical Sciences, University of Nottingham, Nottingham, UK

Udaya S. Tantry, Ph.D. Sinai Center for Thrombosis
Research, Sinai Hospital of Baltimore, Baltimore, MD, USA

Jonathan Watt West of Scotland Regional Heart & Lung
Centre, Golden Jubilee National Hospital,
Glasgow, UK

Daniel M. Witt Department of Pharmacy,
Clinical Pharmacy Research & Applied Pharmacogenomics,
Kaiser Permanente Colorado, Aurora, CO, USA

Chapter 1
Antiplatelet Agents: Current and Novel

Stan Heptinstall

Introduction

Antiplatelet agents are used to reduce platelet function and the contribution of platelets to thrombus formation. As such, antiplatelet agents are used as antithrombotic agents. Ideally they add to the natural mechanisms that are in place to regulate platelet function *in vivo*.

Before looking in some detail at the drugs that are currently in use to help reduce platelet function and the novel agents that are on the horizon, we will start by looking at platelets, what they are and the functions they perform that are relevant to their involvement in thrombosis and also allow them to perform their physiological role in haemostasis.

S. Heptinstall B.Sc., Ph.D.
Division of Cardiovascular Medicine,
School of Clinical Sciences, University of Nottingham,
Nottingham, UK
e-mail: s.heptinstall@nottingham.ac.uk

A. Ferro, D.A. Garcia (eds.), *Antiplatelet and Anticoagulation Therapy*, Current Cardiovascular Therapy,
DOI 10.1007/978-1-4471-4297-3_1,
© Springer-Verlag London 2013

1

TABLE I.I Platelets and their role in health and disease

Platelets	Blood cells involved in haemostasis and thrombosis
Haemostasis	Physiological mechanism for control of bleeding, initiated by formation of a haemostatic plug
Thrombosis	Pathological clot formation leading for example to unstable angina, myocardial infarction and stroke

TABLE 1.2 What are platelets?

	Number	Diameter (μm)
Platelets	150,000–400,000/μl	2
Leucocytes	4,000–11,000/μl	12
Erythrocytes	4,000,000–7,000,000/μl	6

Produced from megakaryocytes in the bone marrow
Normally disc-shaped and dormant
After activation, undergo shape change and become functional

What Are Platelets?

The physiological function of platelets is in haemostasis, the control of bleeding, and people with a low number of platelets and people with severely defective platelet function are at risk of bruising and excessive bleeding following injury. Platelets also have a pathological role in thrombosis (Table 1.1).

Platelets are the smallest of the blood cells. They are disc shaped and are about 2 μm in diameter; their normal number is within the range 150,000–400,000 per μl of blood. This compares with about 8,000 per μl for leucocytes, which are the largest of the blood cells with a diameter of about 12 μm, and 5,000,000 per μl for erythrocytes, with a diameter of about 6 μm (Table 1.2).

Platelets are produced from megakaryocytes in the bone marrow. These grow and develop and then fragment, each megakaryocyte producing many thousands of platelets [1]. These then enter the circulation where they remain for about 10 days before being removed by the reticulo-endothelial system. Production of platelets is under the control of thrombopoietin [2].

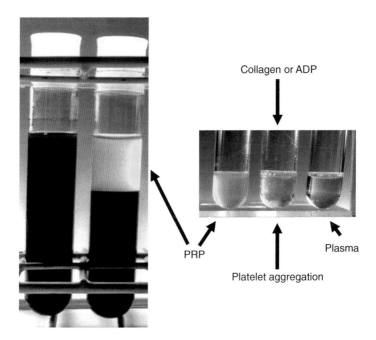

Collagen or ADP

PRP

Plasma

Platelet aggregation

FIGURE 1.1 Platelet aggregation in platelet-rich plasma (PRP)

What Functional Roles Do Platelets Perform?

The main visible example of platelet function is platelet aggregation, which is something that can be observed very easily. If a sample of blood is taken from a volunteer and added to a tube that contains an anticoagulant such as sodium citrate to prevent the blood from clotting, following which the blood is centrifuged at low speed, the larger and denser erythrocytes and leucocytes settle at the bottom of the tube and the smaller and less dense platelets are retained at the top of the tube in the liquid part of the blood, the blood plasma. The upper part is called platelet-rich plasma or PRP. This portion of the blood can be removed and is the starting point for many studies of platelet function (Fig. 1.1).

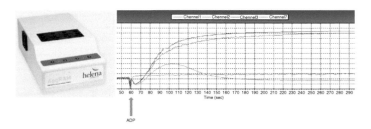

FIGURE 1.2 Platelet aggregation measured by monitoring changes in light transmission

When a small number of collagen fibres or a low concentration of adenosine diphosphate (ADP) is added to the PRP following which the PRP is agitated or stirred, the platelets aggregate together to an extent such that large clumps of platelets can be observed with the naked eye. Indeed this methodology is the basis for the main way in which platelet aggregation is measured, the approach originally used by Gustav Born [3]. Optical aggregometry simply involves measuring the amount of light that can be transmitted through a sample of PRP stirred in an aggregometer. The more light that is transmitted the greater the extent of the platelet aggregation that occurs (Fig. 1.2).

The initial effects of agents such as collagen or ADP on platelets are to bring about a change in shape of the platelets from their normal disc form into a more spherical form on which pseudopodia appear. Such shape-changed platelets immediately start to aggregate together. Subsequently many hundreds of thousands of platelets participate in the platelet aggregates that form [4] (Fig. 1.3).

The main initiators of platelet aggregation and other forms of platelet function that are relevant to the role of platelets in both haemostasis and thrombosis are collagen, thrombin, ADP and thromboxane A_2 (TXA_2) (Table 1.3).

Collagen occupies the space in blood vessels directly beneath the protective layer of endothelial cells and is exposed following damage to the blood vessel through injury. Platelets adhere to collagen and this leads to platelet

Unstimulated platelets   Stimulated platelets

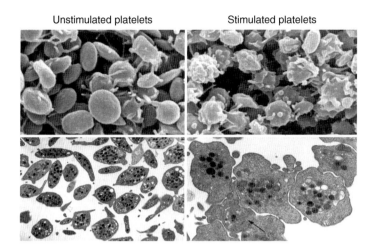

FIGURE 1.3 Scanning (*top*) and transmission (*bottom*) electron micrographs of platelets in PRP before and after stimulation with ADP

TABLE 1.3 Initiators of platelet activation: collagen, thrombin, ADP and TXA_2

- Collagen is exposed following vascular injury or plaque rupture

- Platelets adhere via GPIa/IIa, GPVI, GPIb/VIX-vWF

- Thrombin is generated after tissue factor exposure following vascular injury or plaque rupture and on blood leucocytes

- Thrombin – platelet interaction is via PAR-1 and PAR-4 receptors

- ADP is released from damaged tissues, red cells and platelets and is also derived from ATP via CD39

- ADP interacts with $P2Y_1$ and $P2Y_{12}$ receptors

- TXA_2 is synthesised by platelets

- TXA_2 interacts with TP receptors

activation, subsequent platelet aggregation, and consequent haemostatic plug formation leading to cessation of bleeding from the damaged blood vessel. Platelets also adhere to the collagen that is exposed when an atherosclerotic plaque ruptures. This also leads to platelet activation, subsequent platelet aggregation and, in this case, partial or complete occlusion of the blood vessel giving rise to unstable angina, myocardial infarction or stroke.

Collagen interacts directly with "receptors" for collagen on the surface of platelets [5]. These include a complex of glycoproteins known as GPIa/Ib and also a glycoprotein known as GPVI. Collagen also interacts indirectly with a complex of glycoproteins known as GPIb/V/IX via von-Willebrand factor (vWF), a plasma protein that serves as a link between the collagen and the GPIb/V/IX complex. This mechanism of interaction is of particular relevance where the platelet/collagen interaction occurs in areas of very rapid blood flow, the collagen/vWF serving in a flexible fishing-rod-like way to engage with a platelet that is passing by.

Another process that leads to platelet activation is generation of thrombin following exposure of tissue factor on a damaged blood vessel or within a ruptured atherosclerotic plaque. Tissue factor can also appear on blood cells such as monocytes and neutrophils following platelet-leucocyte conjugate formation (see below). Thrombin is a protease and interacts with protease-activated receptors (PAR receptors) to activate platelets. Those on platelets are mainly PAR-1 and PAR-4. Thrombin, via its protease activity, cleaves off a small part of the receptor exposing a part of the receptor that immediately interacts with itself to bring about platelet activation [6].

ADP is released directly from damaged cells and tissues and in addition is produced from adenosine triphosphate (ATP), also released from damaged cells and tissues including erythrocytes. Breakdown of ATP to ADP occurs through the action of ectonucleotidases such as CD39 present on blood cells and blood vessels. But possibly the main source of the ADP that engages in platelet activation is that derived from the platelets themselves. Both ADP and ATP are secreted from platelet storage granules known as dense bodies following activation by another agent, e.g. collagen or thrombin. In this way the ADP serves to amplify the effects of the primary stimulus. ADP interacts directly with two purinergic receptors known as $P2Y_1$

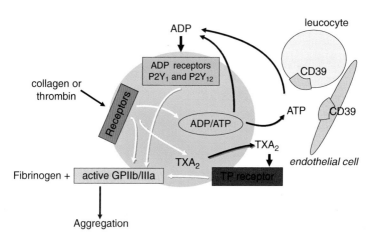

FIGURE 1.4 Agents and receptors involved in platelet activation

and $P2Y_{12}$ and it is the combined effect of ADP at these two receptors that leads to platelet activation [7] (Fig. 1.4).

TXA_2 is another agent that is produced by platelets themselves following primary stimulation by another agent. Arachidonic acid is released from intracellular membranes through the action of a phospholipase and converted first to prostaglandin G_2 and prostaglandin H_2 via a cyclo-oxygenase enzyme and then to TXA_2 via the action of thromboxane synthase. The TXA_2 produced, like ADP, serves to amplify the effects of the primary stimulus. It does so via the TP receptor on the platelet surface [8].

Occupation of a particular receptor on platelets by a particular agent leads to platelet activation. Platelet activation means that a series of inter-related signal transduction events occur within the intracellular region of the cell leading to a functional response, such as aggregation, secretion or TXA_2 synthesis. The events include mobilisation of Ca^{2+} within the cell, phosphoinositide breakdown, phosphorylation of various proteins and enzymes, and alterations in contractile proteins involved in both platelet shape change and secretion. Platelet activation also leads to platelet-leucocyte conjugate

TABLE 1.4 Platelet functional responses that are believed to contribute to haemostasis and thrombosis

- Platelet adhesion to collagen
- Platelet activation by collagen and thrombin
- Platelet aggregation
- Secretion of ADP and ATP
- TXA_2 synthesis
- Expression of P-selection
- Platelet-leucocyte conjugation
- Microparticle formation
- Thrombin/fibrin generation

formation and production of platelet microparticles. There are also changes within the external membrane of platelets associated with creation of a catalytic surface that encourages thrombin formation and subsequent generation of fibrin, the end product of the coagulation cascade [7] (Table 1.4).

An important consequence of platelet activation is a conformational change in a complex of glycoproteins on the surface of platelets known as the GPIIb/IIIa complex, which is essential for platelet aggregation. One of the results of platelet activation is a conformational change in GPIIb/IIIa, which results in the glycoprotein complex being transformed into a receptor for fibrinogen. The latter, a plasma protein that is bivalent (i.e. one end of the molecule is the same as the other), then links a GPIIb/IIIa on one platelet to a GPIIb/IIIa on an adjacent platelet. In total there are some 50,000–100,000 GPIIb/IIIa complexes per platelet so multiple GPIIb/IIIa-fibrinogen-GPIIb/IIIa interactions can occur and this leads to platelet aggregation [9] (Fig. 1.5).

An additional consequence of platelet activation is that a component of the membrane of α – granules in platelets known as P-selectin or CD62P appears on the outer surface of the platelet. This mediates an interaction with leucocytes, particularly monocytes and neutrophils, via P-selectin glycoprotein

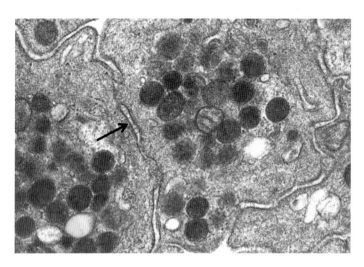

FIGURE 1.5 Platelet aggregation mediated by GPIIb/IIIa and fibrinogen

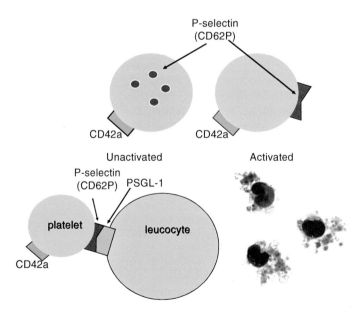

FIGURE 1.6 Generation of P-selectin and platelet-leucocyte conjugates following platelet activation

TABLE 1.5 Factors that contribute to thrombin/fibrin generation

- Tissue factor exposure on damaged blood vessels

- Activated platelets which act as a catalyst of thrombin formation via exposure of negatively charged phospholipids and release of factor V

- Platelet-leucocyte conjugation leading to tissue factor generation

- Platelet microparticles which also act as a catalyst of thrombin formation

ligand 1 (PSGL1) leading to platelet-leucocyte conjugate formation [10] (Fig. 1.6).

Platelets can also break down to smaller particles known as microparticles as a consequence of the activation process [11]. Activated platelets and platelet-leucocyte conjugates and also platelet microparticles provide catalytic surfaces for thrombin generation and consequent generation of fibrin, the end product of the coagulation cascade (Table 1.5).

It is believed that, collectively, all these functional responses contribute both to haemostatic plug formation at points of vascular damage thus fulfilling the physiological role of platelets. They also contribute to the formation of the structures (thrombi) that form on ruptured atherosclerotic plaques that are responsible for partial or complete occlusion of arteries with the clinical consequences of unstable angina, myocardial infarction and stroke. Both haemostatic plugs and thrombi are composed of masses of aggregated platelets together with adherent leucocytes and strands of fibrin (Fig. 1.7).

How Is Platelet Function Suppressed Naturally?

Given that platelets are activated so readily by agents such as collagen, thrombin, ADP and TXA_2 (and also other agents that have not been discussed), perhaps the most remarkable thing is that most of us do not suffer the thrombotic problems that are associated with what platelets do. This is believed to be because of natural control mechanisms that are in place to inhibit platelet function (Table 1.6).

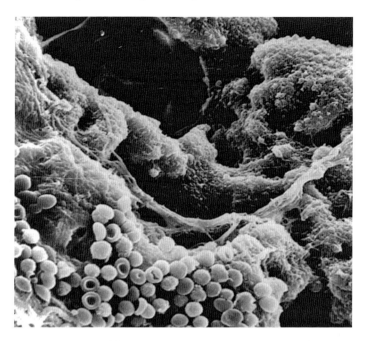

FIGURE 1.7 Thrombi are composed of aggregated platelets with adherent leucocytes and strings of fibrin, the end product of the coagulation cascade

TABLE 1.6 How is platelet function suppressed naturally?

- Prostaglandin I_2 (prostacyclin) produced by intact endothelial cells
- Prostaglandin D_2 and prostaglandin E_1
- Nitric oxide produced by intact endothelial cells
- ADP removal by the ectonucleotidase CD39
- Adenosine?
- Prostaglandin E_2?

Platelet function is inhibited by agents that act directly on platelets to reduce their function and also by the rapid removal of platelet activating agents. Endothelium-derived prostaglandin I_2 (PGI_2, otherwise known as prostacyclin) and nitric oxide (NO) are perhaps the most well known of the agents that act directly on platelets to reduce their function. PGI_2 acts at the IP receptor on the platelet surface, which is linked to the enzyme adenylate cyclase. Occupation of the IP receptor by PGI_2 stimulates adenylate cyclase to convert ATP that is present intracellularly into cyclic adenosine monophosphate (cAMP), which is a potent inhibitor of the signal transduction processes involved in platelet activation referred to earlier [12] (Fig. 1.8).

Similarly, vascular endothelial cells produce NO, which can gain access to the interior of the platelet where it stimulates the enzyme soluble guanylate cyclase to produce cyclic guanosine monophosphate (cGMP), which similarly inhibits platelet function [13] (Fig. 1.9). Indeed, PGI_2 and NO acting together work in a synergistic manner to cause rather profound inhibition of platelet function [14].

As well as PGI_2 there are other prostaglandins produced by vascular and other cells that inhibit platelet function [15] including PGD_2 and PGE_1 which also act by raising cAMP in platelets. PGD_2 acts mainly via the DP receptor on platelets [16] and PGE_1 mainly via the IP receptor [17]. The effect on platelets of another prostaglandin, PGE_2, will be discussed below; PGE_2 is another important prostaglandin in that it derives from atherosclerotic plaque and inflammatory tissue [18].

As stated above, ATP can be converted to ADP and thereby contribute to platelet activation. This conversion is accomplished by the ectonucleotidase CD39 that is present on endothelial cells [19] and also on most blood leucocytes [20, 21]. However, the same CD39 is also able to remove a further phosphate from ADP to produce adenosine monophosphate (AMP), which has no direct effect on platelet function, and thereby removes the potentiating effect of ADP. Presumably the widespread occurrence of CD39 within the blood and vasculature means that this is a major mechanism in the natural control of platelet function [22].

However, further to this, there is widespread availability of the enzyme 5'-nucleotidase on cells and in blood plasma that converts AMP into adenosine, which is interesting because

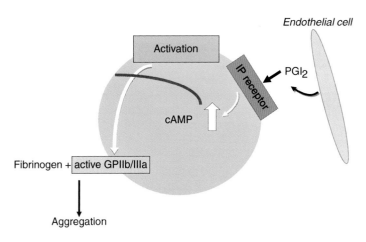

FIGURE 1.8 PGI$_2$: mechanism of action

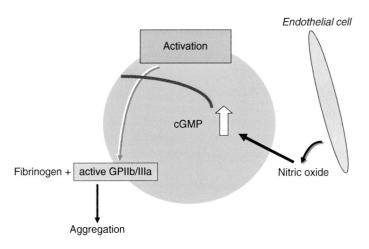

FIGURE 1.9 Nitric oxide: mechanism of action

adenosine, like PGI$_2$, PGD$_2$ and PGE$_1$, is a potent inhibitor of
platelet function, also acting via increasing the concentration
of cAMP in platelets, and in this case acting mainly via the
A$_{2A}$ receptor. Consequently, not only is ADP removed by the
combination of CD39 and 5'-nucleotidase, but also a
potential inhibitor of platelet function is produced. But this

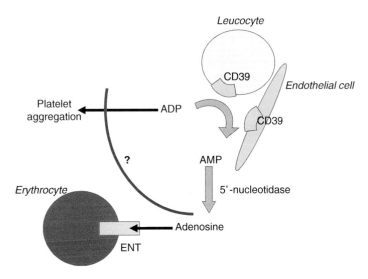

FIGURE 1.10 Inhibition of platelet function by adenosine derived from ADP?

consideration does not stop here. Adenosine produced in blood is rapidly removed via uptake into erythrocytes via the equilibrative nucleoside transporter (ENT), so may not be available to interact with platelets [23, 24]. Thus there is a question mark against the possibility that adenosine derived from ADP really does act as a natural inhibitor of platelet function (Fig. 1.10). Nevertheless, this consideration does have implications for drug therapy as described below.

The other natural prostaglandin against which a question mark exists is PGE_2. This prostaglandin is produced by atherosclerotic plaques and also by inflamed tissue and might be expected to influence platelets in the circulation [18]. The problem here, however, is that PGE_2 has two diametrically opposite effects on platelet function. This is because PGE_2 interacts with two different receptors on platelets, the EP3 receptor and the EP4 receptor [25]. Interaction with the EP4 receptor produces much the same effect as PGI_2 and adenosine, causing an increase in cAMP via stimulation of adenylate

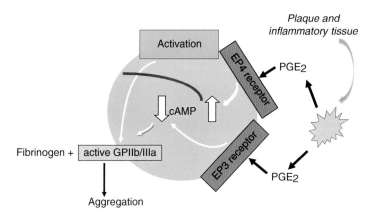

FIGURE 1.11 PGE$_2$: mechanism of action

cyclase. However interaction with the EP3 receptor has the opposite effect. This results in inhibition of adenylate cyclase and a reduction in cAMP leading to promotion of platelet function. This is in the same way that interaction of ADP with the P2Y$_{12}$ receptor causes inhibition of adenylate cyclase and subsequent promotion of platelet function. Consequently PGE$_2$ acting at the EP3 receptor largely cancels out its effect at the EP4 receptor, and indeed net promotion of platelet function has been reported under some experimental circumstances [26]. Consequently PGE$_2$ cannot be regarded as a natural antiplatelet agent (Fig. 1.11). Nevertheless, once again, this particular mechanism of action does have implications for identification of potential antiplatelet drugs, as will be described below.

In completing this section on the natural control of platelet function it is pertinent to point out that TXA$_2$, one of the major agents that promotes platelet function, and also PGI$_2$, one of the major agents that naturally inhibits platelet function, are chemically very unstable and break down within seconds to TXB$_2$ and 6-keto-PGF$_{1\alpha}$ respectively, which have no further effects on platelet function. So, presumably, the impact of both of these agents is very much limited to the points at which they are produced.

TABLE 1.7 Approaches to modulating platelet function

- TXA$_2$ inhibitors (aspirin and other TXA$_2$ inhibitors)
- P2Y$_{12}$ antagonists (clopidogrel, prasugrel, ticagrelor, cangrelor)
- Agents that influence cAMP, cGMP and adenosine metabolism (dipyridamole, cilostazol)
- GPIIb/IIIa antagonists (abciximab, eptifibatide, tirofiban)
- Thrombin antagonists (vorapaxar)
- Collagen antagonists (PR-15)
- EP3 antagonists (DG-041)

Antiplatelet Agents

And so we come to our consideration of the pharmaceutical agents, current and novel, which influence platelet function and are already used, or may be used in the future, as antithrombotic therapy. Clearly, on the basis of the discussion so far, there are many directions in which platelet function can be inhibited. For example, pharmaceutical agents can be (and often have been) identified that prevent the interaction with their receptors of particular agents that activate platelets. Similarly, there are pharmaceutical agents that mimic the effects of natural agents that inhibit platelet function. There are also agents that interfere with one or other of the many intracellular signal transduction processes that are involved in platelet activation. However, there are relatively few drugs that have been identified as being suitable for provision of successful antithrombotic therapy, and it is these that will be the focus of attention here (Table 1.7).

TXA$_2$ Inhibitors

Agents that prevent either TXA$_2$ production in platelets or the action of TXA$_2$ at TP receptors on platelets have been a focus of attention as potential antithrombotic therapy for

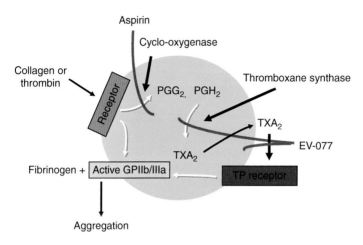

FIGURE 1.12 Inhibition of platelet function by TXA$_2$ inhibitors

many years. The approaches considered are inhibition of the cyclo-oxygenase enzyme in platelets, inhibition of thromboxane synthase, agents that act as antagonists at the TP receptor (so called TXA$_2$ antagonists) and agents that combine some of these properties within one molecule. The agent that has received by far the most attention is aspirin.

Aspirin

Aspirin inhibits the cyclo-oxygenase enzyme in platelets that converts arachidonic acid into the prostaglandin endoperoxides PGG$_2$ and PGH$_2$ and thus what would have been the subsequent conversion of these via thromboxane synthase to TXA$_2$ [27] (Fig. 1.12). Through this mechanism aspirin inhibits platelet function in experiments performed wholly *in vitro* (e.g. collagen-induced platelet aggregation is inhibited after adding aspirin to samples of PRP). Also platelet function is inhibited *in vivo* after administration of aspirin to man. The inhibitory effect of aspirin is irreversible. Aspirin is acetylsalicylic acid and the acetyl part of the molecule is transferred to the cyclo-oxygenase rendering the enzyme inactive. Thus the

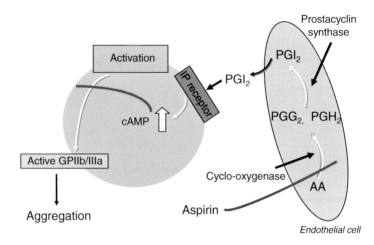

FIGURE 1.13 Inhibition of vascular prostaglandin synthesis by aspirin

in vivo effects of aspirin are evident for the lifetime of the platelets that are affected. Thus for newly formed platelets in the circulation its effects are present for about 10 days.

Conventionally it is "low-dose" aspirin (a dose of around 75 mg/day) that is administered orally once a day as anti-thrombotic therapy, which is all that is needed for near-complete inhibition of TXA_2 synthesis and platelet function [28, 29]. But there is another reason for using such a low dose. Prostaglandins such as PGI_2 are considered to be important in the natural control of platelet function, and PGI_2, and indeed all other prostaglandins, are synthesised in much the same way as TXA_2. In all cases a cyclo-oxygenase converts a liberated fatty acid (usually arachidonic acid) into prosta-glandin endoperoxides, which are then selectively converted into the final product. The enzyme that converts the PGG_2 and PGH_2 into PGI_2 is prostacyclin synthase. Aspirin is just as capable of inhibiting the cyclo-oxygenase in endothelial cells and thereby PGI_2 synthesis as it is of inhibiting the cyclo-oxygenase in platelets and thereby TXA_2 synthesis, which would not be ideal (Fig. 1.13) [27].

However, once administered, aspirin is very rapidly metab-olised, and because newly administered aspirin interacts with platelets early (in the portal circulation), low doses of the drug interact preferentially with platelets and inhibit TXA_2 synthesis in preference to PGI_2 synthesis. In contrast, high doses can interfere with both synthesis of TXA_2 in platelets and synthesis of PGI_2 (and other prostaglandins) in the vasculature.

It was the ISIS-2 trial [30] that brought the use of aspirin to the fore. In this study the beneficial effects of low dose aspirin, streptokinase and low dose aspirin in combination with streptokinase were compared with placebo in patients with a recent myocardial infarction, and it was clearly demonstrated that all three treatments produced clinical benefit. Also, the meta-analyses of trials of aspirin as antithrombotic therapy produced by the Antiplatelet Trialists' Collaboration and the Antithrombotic Trialists' Collaboration were hugely influential in ensuring its use in a wide-variety of patients at-risk of thrombotic events [31–33]. Aspirin is the most widely used antithrombotic agent worldwide.

Other TXA_2 Inhibitors

Over the years there has been a considerable focus on agents that act as inhibitors of thromboxane synthase (e.g. daxoxiben [34]), agents that act as TXA_2 antagonists (e.g. sulotroban [35]), and combination agents that combine both of these activities (e.g. picotamide [36]). All of these received a great deal of attention by researchers as agents to be used in place of aspirin as antithrombotic agents but none of them completed the development programme. However there is currently a resurgence of interest in this area through the emergence of a new combination agent known as EV-077 [37]. This drug is currently undergoing investigation as an agent to reduce complications in diabetic patients.

$P2Y_{12}$ Antagonists

Agents that act as antagonists of the effects of ADP at the $P2Y_{12}$ receptor on platelets are a major focus as antithrombotic agents (Table 1.8). One agent (clopidogrel) is already in

TABLE 1.8 Differences between $P2Y_{12}$ antagonists

Drug	Action	Reversibility	Onset	offset	Inhibition of platelet function	Variability of effect
Clopidogrel	Prodrug	Irreversible	Slow	Slow	Partial	Variable
Prasugrel	Prodrug	Irreversible	Fast	Slow	More complete	Less variable
Ticagrelor[a]	Direct	Reversible	Fast	Faster	More complete	Less variable
Cangrelor[b]	Direct	Reversible	Immediate	Very rapid	More complete	Less variable

[a]Significant effect on mortality in PLATO
[b]Clinical trials still incomplete

widespread use, two new agents (prasugrel and ticagrelor) are available as alternatives for use in place of clopidogrel, and another agent (cangrelor) is also on the horizon.

Clopidogrel

Clopidogrel is a drug that inhibits ADP-induced platelet aggregation *in vivo* following administration to man. It belongs to a class of drugs known as thienopyridines. It is pro-drug, which means that it has to be converted into an active metabolite for its effects to be seen, and therefore does not affect platelet function when added to blood or PRP *in vitro*. Its active metabolite is an agent that interacts with the $P2Y_{12}$ receptor on platelets and thereby renders it incapable of interacting with ADP. As mentioned above, ADP activates platelets via two purinergic receptors on platelets, the $P2Y_1$ receptor and the $P2Y_{12}$ receptor. In fact, both receptors need to be occupied by ADP for a full platelet response, and in the absence of $P2Y_{12}$ the effect of ADP on platelet function is much weaker than in its presence. For example, following effective $P2Y_{12}$ blockade the aggregation that is brought about when a high concentration of ADP is added to PRP is weak and the aggregates soon start to come apart, or disag-gregate, following the initial stimulus. Clopidogrel's active metabolite interacts with the $P2Y_{12}$ receptor covalently and irreversibly via certain sulphydryl groups on the receptor. So, like aspirin, its effects are evident for the lifetime of the affected platelets, which, for newly formed platelets, is about 10 days [7].

Clopidogrel is conventionally administered orally at a "maintenance dose" of 75 mg/day although the first dose administered, the "loading dose", can be higher e.g. 300 or 600 mg. The use of a higher loading dose is in an attempt to produce inhibition of platelet function as quickly as possible in severely ill people. Nevertheless, the rate of onset of inhibition is still quite slow whatever the initial dose of clopidogrel used, and also the overall degree of inhibition of platelet function

achieved is lower than that obtained with other $P2Y_{12}$ antagonists (see below). Also, the extent of the inhibitory effects of
clopidogrel is very different in different people, which is related
to differences in the amount of active metabolite generated. This
is in part determined by genetic differences including a
reduced function allele of the CYP2C19 gene. This is important because people with high residual platelet function while
on clopidogrel are more likely to experience thrombotic
events than those with low residual platelet function [38].

Clopidogrel was not the first thienopyridine to be used as an
antithrombotic agent. This drug replaced a previous drug
called ticlopidine, which, despite providing clear inhibition of
ADP-induced platelet aggregation following administration to
man, turned out to have some unwanted side-effects, particularly transient neutropenia in some patients. Clopidogrel
became the replacement for ticlopidine when it was found to
not have the same side effects [39]. Clopidogrel came of age
when it was compared with low-dose aspirin in the CAPRIE
trial and found to provide a marginally better antithrombotic
effect than aspirin [40]. Also, this trial clearly established the
clinical value of the use of a $P2Y_{12}$ antagonist as antithrombotic
therapy and that the strategy of reducing the ADP-induced
platelet function was as good or better than blocking TXA_2
synthesis in platelets. The trials that followed CAPRIE were
designed to answer the question, would clopidogrel in combination with low-dose aspirin provide better antithrombotic
therapy than aspirin alone, and it was the success of these further trials that led to the widespread use of clopidogrel together
with aspirin in people at-risk of coronary thrombosis. In contrast current recommendations are that clopidogrel should be
used alone in patients with a previous stroke since no clear
benefit of using the two drugs in combination has emerged.

Prasugrel

Prasugrel is also a thienopyridine and is remarkably similar
to clopidogrel in many ways. Like clopidogrel, prasugrel is a
pro-drug and depends on its active metabolite for its antiplatelet effect. Like clopidogrel, its effect is via a covalent

irreversible interaction with the $P2Y_{12}$ receptor and consequent inhibition of ADP-induced platelet function. Indeed, experiments performed *in vitro* in which the effects of the active metabolites of clopidogrel and prasugrel are compared indicate little if any difference between them. However, prasugrel does differ from clopidogrel in one important regard; its active metabolite is produced in one metabolic step rather than two, and the effects of this are more rapid inhibition of platelet function following administration, more intense inhibition at the dose at which it is administered, and much less variability in the degree of inhibition seen in different people. Also the doses needed are smaller than those for clopidogrel. Prasugrel is currently administered orally at a dose of 10 mg/day following a 60 mg loading dose [7].

The main clinical trial that established prasugrel as a real competitor to clopidogrel was the TRITON-TIMI 38 trial [41]. This compared prasugrel taken with low-dose aspirin to clopidogrel taken with low-dose aspirin in patients with acute coronary syndromes (ACS) who were scheduled for percutaneous coronary intervention (PCI). In this trial prasugrel significantly reduced the main outcome measure, which was a composite of vascular death, myocardial infarction and stroke, but at the expense of some increase in major bleeding. At that time some increase in major bleeding was thought to be an inevitable consequence of more effective antiplatelet therapy given the role of platelets in haemostasis, but more on this below. Prasugrel is now licensed for use in patients with ACS undergoing PCI [42].

Ticagrelor

Like clopidogrel and prasugrel, ticagrelor is also a $P2Y_{12}$ antagonist but it does differ from these other drugs in several regards [43]. Ticagrelor belongs to a different class of chemical structures. It is a cyclopentyl-triazolo-pyrimidine; the drug was formerly known as AZD6140. Ticagrelor is a drug that acts directly at the $P2Y_{12}$ receptor to inhibit ADP-induced platelet function. It does not compete directly with ADP at the ADP binding site but occupies an adjacent binding site and acts as an allosteric modulator resulting in a conformational change of the receptor rendering it incapable of interacting with ADP [44]. Unlike clopidogrel and prasugrel the inhibition is reversible rather than irreversible, which means that the drug can come off the receptor when treatment is curtailed and platelet function can be restored. However, in actuality, this reversal of inhibition is quite slow (see below). Like clopidogrel and prasugrel, ticagrelor does have an active metabolite but this is present in lower quantities than the parent drug and it appears to act in an identical manner to the parent drug [45].

There have been a number of studies in which the pharmacological effects of ticagrelor have been compared with those of clopidogrel. These include DISPERSE [46] and DISPERSE2 [47], the ONSET/OFFSET study [48] and the RESPOND study [49]. Also pharmacological data were obtained in a large clinical intervention study called PLATO [50]. Collectively these studies demonstrated that ticagrelor taken orally at its currently recommended dose (180 mg loading dose and 90 mg twice daily as maintenance therapy) compared with clopidogrel taken as currently recommended, provided more rapid inhibition of ADP-induced platelet function following initial administration, more intense inhibition that remained high between consecutive doses of the drug, and, as described above for prasugrel, much less variability in the degree of inhibition seen in different people. Ticagrelor also added to the inhibition of aggregation in patients who were started on ticagrelor immediately after stopping clopidogrel. On cessation of drug administration it still took several days for the inhibitory effect on platelet function to disappear despite ticagrelor's reversible mode of action, but this did occur more quickly than with clopidogrel with baseline levels achieved after 5 days rather than 7 days.

PLATO [51, 52] was the study that led to ticagrelor being licensed as an alternative to clopidogrel in a wide range of patients with acute coronary syndromes. Remarkably, ticagrelor taken with aspirin not only proved to be superior to clopidogrel taken with aspirin in reducing a composite endpoint of death from vascular causes, myocardial infarction and stroke, it also reduced overall mortality. Also this was achieved without a marked increase in major bleeding, which no one can really understand given the more effective inhibition of platelet function that was achieved. A negative side effect was an increased incidence of dyspnoea in the ticagrelor-treated patients. In this international study there was also a geographical anomaly that warrants mention. There was one world region in which the antithrombotic advantage achieved with ticagrelor was not seen; this was in North America.

There are several questions thrown up through the PLATO trial. Why was a benefit evident that has not been seen in other trials in which effective $P2Y_{12}$ antagonism was achieved, e.g. TRITON TIMI 38? Why was major bleeding not greater than might have been predicted in the PLATO trial? Why did dyspnoea occur in some patients? What is the nature of the North American paradox? No clear answers to these questions have emerged.

Although ticagrelor inhibits effects of ADP at the $P2Y_{12}$ receptor in an allosteric way, which is different to the way in which other $P2Y_{12}$ antagonists interact with the receptor, the effects on platelet function of the different drugs appear to be the same [53]. It is speculated that the occurrence of dyspnoea may be related to accumulation of adenosine following an effect of ticagrelor on adenosine uptake into erythrocytes [54]. If this were the case there could be further implications in that accumulating adenosine might be expected to have other consequences. And indeed there is some experimental evidence to demonstrate an effect of accumulating adenosine on coronary blood flow in the presence of ticagrelor [55]. On the other hand, others have not been able to detect any effect of adenosine derived from ADP on platelet function in intact blood in the presence of ticagrelor or any other $P2Y_{12}$ antagonist tested, despite performing careful experiments to look at that possibility, and despite obtaining positive results in the presence of dipyridamole, which is a well-known inhibitor of adenosine uptake [56].

Regarding the North American paradox, one difference that emerged between North America and the rest of the world when examining the fine detail of local practice was that the low-dose aspirin used in North America (around 300 mg/day) is higher than that elsewhere, and the possibility is discussed that this is part of the problem [57]. Interestingly, it is now becoming very clear that there is good synergism between the inhibitory effects of a $P2Y_{12}$ antagonist and any agent that inhibits platelet function via an effect on cAMP [58–60]. So the possibility exists that higher doses of aspirin, through inhibition of synthesis of vascular prostaglandins that act as natural inhibitors of platelet function by increasing cAMP, may have interfered with this synergism, and that this is part of the explanation of the North American paradox. The concept of synergism between a $P2Y_{12}$ antagonist and an agent such as PGI_2 is illustrated diagrammatically in Fig. 1.14.

Interestingly, when the Food and Drug Administration in the USA granted a licence it came with a warning that co-use of aspirin at doses greater than 100 mg/day may reduce

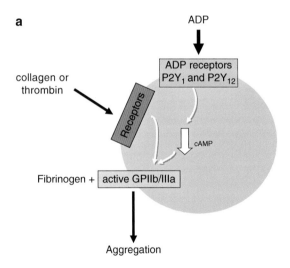

FIGURE 1.14 (a) ADP lowers cAMP and promotes platelet function; (b) PGI_2 counters the effect of ADP on cAMP; (c) a $P2Y_{12}$ antagonist prevents ADP lowering cAMP allowing PGI_2 to provide very effective inhibition of platelet function; (d) if aspirin blocks PGI_2 synthesis, cAMP is unable to contribute to inhibition of platelet function

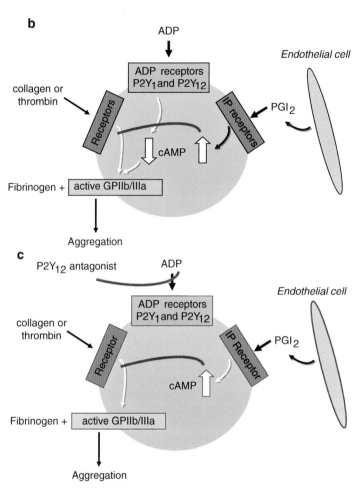

FIGURE 1.14 (continued)

d

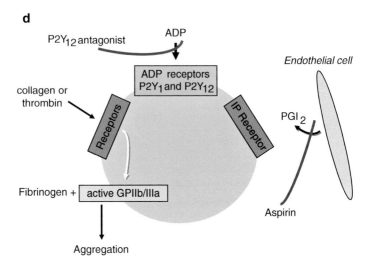

FIGURE 1.14 (continued)

ticagrelor's effectiveness. Also, the manufacturers were required to engage in education programmes aimed at physicians to alert them about the risk of using higher doses of aspirin. Ticagrelor also needs to be dispensed with a Medication Guide that is to be distributed each time a patient fills their prescription [61, 62].

Cangrelor

The $P2Y_{12}$ antagonists discussed so far are the only ones that are currently licensed for use as antithrombotic therapy, however another $P2Y_{12}$ antagonist, cangrelor, is also in development.

Cangrelor is a $P2Y_{12}$ antagonist that was known previously as AR-C69931 and as such received a great deal of attention from scientists interested in the $P2Y_{12}$ receptor and its role in platelet function, and there are a huge number of scientific papers in which the drug has been used experimentally.

Cangrelor is the perfect drug for experimental investigations. It is water soluble, and acts directly and immediately to inhibit ADP-induced platelet function when added to blood or PRP *in vitro*. It is stable and potent. It is selective as a $P2Y_{12}$ antagonist [53] despite one paper to the contrary [63]. Like ticagrelor it is a reversible inhibitor of platelet function, but unlike ticagrelor it comes off the receptor within minutes of the drug being discontinued [64].

Cangrelor is being developed as a drug for intravenous rather than oral use. It may be a particularly useful where the presence of a $P2Y_{12}$ antagonist is required during clinical procedures where there is a risk of bleeding [65]. Because of its highly reversible nature, cessation of infusion allows full platelet activity to return very quickly. There is an issue, though, about changing treatments from cangrelor to clopidogrel or prasugrel because it has been shown that cangrelor can interfere with the ability of the active metabolites of clopidogrel and prasugrel to inhibit ADP-induced platelet function [66, 67].

Elinogrel is another direct-acting and reversible $P2Y_{12}$ antagonist that was in development. Apparently, unlike its competitors, it was to be made available in both intravenous and oral forms [68]. However elinogrel was unexpectedly withdrawn from development in 2012.

Agents That Influence cAMP, cGMP and Adenosine Metabolism

The important roles of natural agents that increase cAMP and cGMP in platelets in the natural control of platelet function have already been discussed. Also discussed is the question mark over the role of adenosine as a natural modulator of platelet function given its rapid removal from blood plasma through uptake into erythrocytes via the equilibrative nucleoside transporter. Dipyridamole and cilostazol are two agents that are in clinical use whose mode of action impacts on cyclic nucleotides and adenosine metabolism.

Dipyridamole and Cilostazol

Dipyridamole is an old drug that was found to inhibit thrombus formation in experimental animals. Subsequently it was shown to have inhibitory effects on platelet function and also to be an inhibitor of adenosine uptake into erythrocytes. It is an inhibitor of phosphodiesterase enzymes. In particular it inhibits the breakdown of cGMP in platelets (and other cells) to GMP. Since cGMP is associated with inhibition of platelet function it is considered that inhibiting the breakdown of this cyclic nucleotide is one of the mechanisms through which platelet function is inhibited. There is also an interaction with nitric oxide, which promotes cGMP production in platelets [69]. In addition dipyridamole is an inhibitor of adenosine uptake into erythrocytes and this is another means through which dipyridamole can affect platelet function [70]. In the section above on natural modulators of platelet function, doubt was expressed as to whether adenosine does act as a natural modulator due to its rapid uptake into erythrocytes. Clearly, adenosine produced in the presence of dipyridamole acting as an inhibitor of adenosine uptake would create an ideal way in which the natural inhibitory effects of adenosine can be utilised (Fig. 1.15).

The ability of adenosine, produced through breakdown of ADP, to inhibit platelet aggregation in the presence of dipyridamole, is markedly amplified when a $P2Y_{12}$ antagonist is also present [60]. Until now, the potential benefits of the combination of a $P2Y_{12}$ antagonist and dipyridamole used in combination as antithrombotic therapy have not been fully understood and further research in this area is needed.

Dipyridamole is a drug that has been, and is still, used extensively in patients with prior stroke.

It is a vasodilator so its use can be accompanied by headache in some patients. Its use as an antithrombotic agent in stroke when used in combination with aspirin was established by the ESPS2 Study [71].

Another drug with a pharmacological profile similar to that of dipyridamole is cilostazol [72]. This also combines

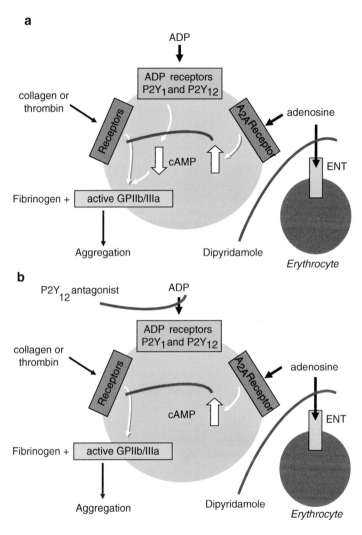

FIGURE 1.15 (**a**) Adenosine generated in the presence of dipyridamole counters the effect of ADP on cAMP; (**b**) a P2Y$_{12}$ antagonist prevents ADP lowering cAMP allowing adenosine to provide very effective inhibition of platelet function

inhibition of a phosphodiesterase enzyme with the ability to inhibit adenosine uptake. This particular drug is used in some patients with peripheral vascular disease and has been shown to increase walking distance.

GPIIb/IIIa Antagonists

As will have become very clear from the discussion on platelet function above, the GPIIb/IIIa complex on platelets is intimately involved in platelet aggregation. GPIIb/IIIa changes its conformation following platelet activation, becomes a receptor for fibrinogen, and the fibrinogen links adjacent platelets together. The GPIIb/IIIa antagonists block the interaction of fibrinogen with the activated GPIIb/IIIa complex. Such drugs do not prevent the initial activation of platelets by the various agents that bring this about, but block what is called "the final common pathway" in the aggregation process. [73].

There are a number of GPIIb/IIIa antagonists that have become available and all have proved to be very effective inhibitors of the platelet aggregation induced by a wide variety of agents.

The drugs available include abciximab, eptifibatide, and tirofiban. Following positive results in clinical trials in which they were administered intravenously during some cardiac interventions, these agents are now used as adjunctive therapy by some cardiac surgeons as a means of preventing the build up of platelets during PCI. Interestingly the separate development of GPIIb/IIIa antagonists to be used as oral medicines in much the same way as the $P2Y_{12}$ antagonists was terminated when clinical trials of such agents resulted in significantly increased mortality. No one understands the reason for this [73].

GPIIb/IIIa antagonists do not prevent platelet activation, they only prevent platelet aggregation. Indeed it has been demonstrated that GPIIb/IIIa antagonists increase platelet-leucocyte conjugate formation [74, 75]. This is a consequence of activated platelets exposing P-selectin and then interacting with blood leucocytes rather than with other platelets in the blood. Platelet-leucocyte conjugates, as well as platelet aggregates, are believed to contribute to thrombus formation and potentially this could be one explanation for the lack of success seen with the oral GPIIb/IIIa antagonists used as antithrombotic drugs.

Thrombin Antagonists

There is no doubt that thrombin plays in important role in thrombus formation. As discussed above, it activates platelets directly mainly via the PAR-1 receptor. In addition thrombin acts to convert fibrinogen to fibrin, the end product of the coagulation cascade, and fibrin is an important component of thrombus. Thrombin production can be reduced through the use of anticoagulants and there is separate interest in the use of such thrombin inhibitors as antithrombotic therapy. But also the effects of thrombin at the PAR-1 receptor can be blocked using a thrombin antagonist such as vorapaxar.

Until quite recently, the concept of using a thrombin antagonist such as vorapaxar as an adjunct to antithrombotic therapy presented an exciting new approach to inhibiting platelet function. Unfortunately, however, a major clinical trial in which vorapaxar was used in addition to standard therapy in patients with ACS had to be terminated prematurely because of an unacceptable increase in major bleeding in the treated patients [76]. So at this point the future of this approach is uncertain.

Collagen Antagonists

Given the importance of collagen in initiating platelet function the concept of blocking the interaction of collagen and platelets is also an important possibility. Perhaps the most advanced of several reported approaches is via the use of a fusion protein known as PR-15 or Revacept. This agent specifically blocks the interaction of collagen with GPVI on platelets and the results of a phase 1 study in which Revacept was infused intravenously into healthy humans has just been

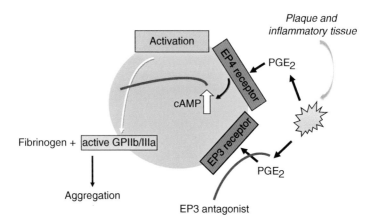

FIGURE 1.16 Inhibition of platelet function by PGE_2 in the presence of an EP3 antagonist

published in which inhibition of collagen-induced platelet aggregation *in vivo* occurred with no apparent negative outcomes, including no increase in measurements of bleeding time [77]. Other collagen antagonists that interfere with the interaction of collagen/vWF with the GPIb/V/IX complex are of interest to investigators but appear to be at an earlier stage in development [78].

EP3 Antagonists

As explained above PGE_2 is produced by atherosclerotic plaques and inflamed tissue and interacts with platelets in two ways. It promotes platelet function through interaction with the EP3 receptor and inhibits platelet function through interaction with the EP4 receptor, and the overall effect depends on the balance between these two interactions (Fig. 1.16).

Against this background emerged the concept of the potential of a drug that acts as an antagonist at EP3 receptors leaving naturally produced PGE_2 to interact with the EP4 receptor only and thereby to inhibit platelet function.

The agent that has been used to study this concept is DG-041, and certainly this agent enables PGE_2 to inhibit platelet function both when added to blood or PRP *in vitro* and *ex vivo* after administration to man [79]. It also adds to the effects of clopidogrel and aspirin when these are co-administered with DG-041 without any effect on bleeding time measurements [80, 81]. It will be interesting to see how far this particular concept is developed in the future.

Key Points

1. Antiplatelet agents are drugs that reduce the ability of platelets to engage in thrombus formation. They do so by reducing the ability of platelets to aggregate together and also by inhibiting other aspects of platelet function.
2. There are several different approaches to inhibiting platelet function and many different types of antiplatelet agents.
3. Some antiplatelet agents are already in clinical use as anti-thrombotic therapy, others are in development.
4. One of the main thromboxane A_2 inhibitors is aspirin, an inhibitor of the cyclo-oxygenase enzyme; it is used in low doses so as to avoid inhibition of synthesis of prostaglandins that serve as natural inhibitors of platelet function.
5. Clopidogrel, prasugrel and ticagrelor are $P2Y_{12}$ antagonists that are already licensed for use, and another agent cangrelor is in development. All these agents differ from each other in several respects and these differences are discussed.
6. Dipyridamole and cilostazol are agents that act via effects on cyclic nucleotides and adenosine metabolism. Their potential use in combination with a $P2Y_{12}$ antagonist should be considered.
7. Some GPIIb/IIIa antagonists are used and are effective intravenously but oral agents are no longer in development.
8. A thrombin antagonist that acts at the PAR-1 receptor was recently shown to enhance bleeding risk to an unacceptable extent and its future development is under review.

9. Collagen antagonists are an interesting approach to anti-thrombotic therapy but are not yet available for clinical use.
10. Agents that act as antagonists at the EP3 receptor on platelets provide a potential new approach to antithrombotic therapy.

Conflicts of Interest   Stan Heptinstall on behalf of the University of Nottingham has received research grants for laboratory investigations on the P2Y$_{12}$ antagonists clopidogrel, prasugrel, ticagrelor and cangrelor and the EP3 antagonist DG-041. He is also a shareholder and director of Platelet Solutions Ltd, a spinout company of the University of Nottingham that engages in platelet function testing.

Acknowledgements   The electron micrographs in Figs. 1.3, 1.5 and 1.7 were produced by Dr. MW Ramsey when he was a medical student at the University of Nottingham.

References

1. Patel SR, Hartwig JH, Italiano Jr JE. The biogenesis of platelets from megakaryocyte proplatelets. J Clin Invest. 2005;115:3348–54.
2. Kuter DJ. Biology and chemistry of thrombopoietic agents. Semin Hematol. 2010;47:243–8.
3. Born GVR. Aggregation of blood platelets by adenosine diphosphate and its reversal. Nature. 1962;194:927–9.
4. Packham MA, Rand ML. Historical perspective on ADP-induced platelet activation. Purinergic Signal. 2011;7:283–92.
5. Varga-Szabo D, Pleines I, Nieswandt B. Cell adhesion mechanisms in platelets. Arterioscler Thromb Vasc Biol. 2008;28:403–12.
6. Leger AJ, Covic L, Kuliopulos A. Protease-activated receptors in cardiovascular diseases. Circulation. 2006;114:1070–7.
7. Wijeyeratne YD, Heptinstall S. Anti-platelet therapy: ADP receptor antagonists. J Clin Pharmacol. 2011;72:647–57.
8. Giannarelli C, Zafar MU, Badimon JJ. Prostanoid and TP-receptors in atherothrombosis: is there a role for their antagonism? Thromb Haemost. 2010;104:949–54.
9. Bennett JS, Berger BW, Billings PC. The structure and function of platelet integrins. J Thromb Haemost. 2009;Suppl 1:200–5.

10. Cerletti C, Tamburrelli C, Izzi B, Gianfagna F, de Gaetano G. Platelet-leukocyte interactions in thrombosis. Thromb Res. 2012;129:263–6.
11. Owens 3rd AP, Mackman N. Microparticles in hemostasis and thrombosis. Circ Res. 2011;108:1284–97.
12. Midgett C, Stitham J, Martin KA, Hwa J. Prostacyclin receptor regulation–from transcription to trafficking. Curr Mol Med. 2011;11:517–28.
13. Truss NJ, Warner TD. Gasotransmitters and platelets. Pharmacol Ther. 2011;132:196–203.
14. Mitchell JA, Ali F, Bailey L, Moreno L, Harrington LS. Role of nitric oxide and prostacyclin as vasoactive hormones released by the endothelium. Exp Physiol. 2008;93:141–7.
15. Whittle BJ, Moncada S, Vane JR. Comparison of the effects of prostacyclin (PGI2), prostaglandin E1 and D2 on platelet aggregation in different species. Prostaglandins. 1978;3:373–8.
16. Giles H, Leff P, Bolofo ML, Kelly MG, Robertson AD. The classification of prostaglandin DP-receptors in platelets and vasculature using BW A868C, a novel, selective and potent competitive antagonist. Br J Pharmacol. 1989;96:291–300.
17. Iyú D, Jüttner M, Glenn JR, White AE, Johnson AJ, Fox SC, Heptinstall S. PGE1 and PGE2 modify platelet function through different prostanoid receptors. Prostaglandins Other Lipid Mediat. 2011;94:9–16.
18. Gross S, Tilly P, Hentsch D, Vonesch JL, Fabre JE. Vascular wall-produced prostaglandin E2 exacerbates arterial thrombosis and atherothrombosis through platelet EP3 receptors. J Exp Med. 2007;204:311–20.
19. Marcus AJ, Broekman MJ, Drosopoulos JHF, Islam N, Alyonycheva TN, Saffer LB, Hajjar KA, Posnett DN, Schoenborn MA, Schooley KA, Gayle RB, Maliszewski CR. The endothelial cells ecto-ADPase responsible for inhibition of platelet function is CD39. J Clin Invest. 1997;99:1351–60.
20. Glenn JR, White AE, Johnson AJ, Fox SC, Behan MWH, Dolan G, Heptinstall S. Leukocyte count and leukocyte ecto-nucleotidase are major determinants of the effects of adenosine triphosphate and adenosine diphosphate on platelet aggregation in human blood. Platelets. 2005;16:159–70.
21. Glenn JR, White AE, Johnson AJ, Fox SC, Myers B, Heptinstall S. Raised levels of CD39 in leucocytosis result in marked inhibition of ADP-induced aggregation via rapid hydrolysis. Platelets. 2008;19:59–69.

38   S. Heptinstall

22. Heptinstall S, Johnson A, Glenn JR, White AE. Adenine nucleotide metabolism in human blood - important roles for leukocytes and erythrocytes. J Thromb Haemost. 2005;3:2331–9.
23. Griffith DA, Jarvis SM. Nucleoside and nucleobase transport systems of mammalian cells. Biochim Biophys Acta. 1996; 1286:153–81.
24. Loffler M, Morote-Garcia JC, Eltzschig SA, Coe IR, Eltzschig HK. Physiological roles of vascular nucleoside transporters. Arterioscler Thromb Vasc Biol. 2007;27:1004–13.
25. Iyú D, Glenn JR, White AE, Johnson AJ, Fox SC, Heptinstall S. The role of prostanoid receptors in mediating the effects of PGE(2) on human platelet function. Platelets. 2010;21:329–42.
26. Gray SJ, Heptinstall S. Interactions between prostaglandin E2 and inhibitors of platelet aggregation which act through cyclic AMP. Eur J Pharmacol. 1991;194:63–70.
27. Botting RM. Inhibitors of cyclooxygenases: mechanisms, selectivity and uses. J Physiol Pharmacol. 2006;57 Suppl 5:113–24.
28. May JA, Heptinstall S, Cole AT, Hawkey CJ. Platelet responses to several agonists and combinations of agonists in whole blood: a placebo controlled comparison of the effects of a once daily dose of plain aspirin 300 mg, plain aspirin 75 mg and enteric coated aspirin 300 mg, in man. Thromb Res. 1997;88:183–92.
29. Perneby C, Wallén NH, Rooney C, Fitzgerald D, Hjemdahl P. Dose- and time-dependent antiplatelet effects of aspirin. Thromb Haemost. 2006;95:652–8.
30. ISIS-2 (Second International Study of Infarct Survival) Collaborative Group. Randomised trial of intravenous streptokinase, oral aspirin, both, or neither among 17,187 cases of suspected acute myocardial infarction: ISIS-2. Lancet. 1988;13 (2(8607)):349–60.
31. Antiplatelet Trialists' Collaboration. Secondary prevention of vascular disease by prolonged antiplatelet treatment. Br Med J. 1988;296:320–31.
32. Antiplatelet Trialists' Collaboration. Collaborative overview of randomised trials of antiplatelet therapy–I: prevention of death, myocardial infarction, and stroke by prolonged antiplatelet therapy in various categories of patients. Br Med J. 1994; 308:81–106.
33. Antithrombotic Trialists' Collaboration. Collaborative meta-analysis of randomised trials of antiplatelet therapy for prevention of death, myocardial infarction, and stroke in high risk patients. Br Med J. 2002;324:71–86.

34. Jones EW, Cockbill SR, Cowley AJ, Hanley SP, Heptinstall S. Effects of dazoxiben and low-dose aspirin on platelet behaviour in man. Br J Clin Pharmacol. 1983;15 Suppl 1:39S–44.
35. Lonsdale RJ, Heptinstall S, Westby JC, Berridge DC, Wenham PW, Hopkinson BR, Makin GS. A study of the use of the thromboxane A2 antagonist, sulotroban, in combination with streptokinase for local thrombolysis in patients with recent peripheral arterial occlusions: clinical effects, platelet function and fibrinolytic parameters. Thromb Haemost. 1993;69:103–11.
36. Pulcinelli FM, Pignatelli P, Pesciotti M, Sebastiani S, Parisi S, Gazzaniga PP. Mechanism of the persisting TxA2 receptor antagonism by picotamide. Thromb Res. 1997;85:207–15.
37. Fontana P, Alberts P, Sakariassen KS, Bounameaux H, Meyer JP, Santana Sorensen A. The dual thromboxane receptor antagonist and thromboxane synthase inhibitor EV-077 is a more potent inhibitor of platelet function than aspirin. J Thromb Haemost. 2011;9:2109–11.
38. Sofi F, Marcucci R, Gori AM, Giusti B, Abbate R, Gensini GF. Clopidogrel non-responsiveness and risk of cardiovascular morbidity. An updated meta-analysis. Thromb Haemost. 2010;103:841–8.
39. Savi P, Herbert JM. Clopidogrel and ticlopidine: P2Y12 adenosine diphosphate-receptor antagonists for the prevention of atherothrombosis. Semin Thromb Hemost. 2005;31:174–83.
40. CAPRIE Steering Committee. A randomised, blinded, trial of clopidogrel versus aspirin in patients at risk of ischaemic events (CAPRIE). Lancet. 1996;348:1329–39.
41. Wiviott SD, Braunwald E, McCabe CH, Montalescot G, Ruzyllo W, Gottlieb S, Neumann FJ, Ardissino D, De Servi S, Murphy SA, Riesmeyer J, Weerakkody G, Gibson CM, Antman EM, TRITON-TIMI 38 Investigators. Prasugrel versus clopidogrel in patients with acute coronary syndromes. N Engl J Med. 2007;357:2001–15.
42. NICE. Prasugrel for the treatment of acute coronary syndromes with percutaneous coronary intervention. 2009. http://www.nice.org.uk/nicemedia/live/12324/45849/45849.pdf Accessed 1 Jan 2012.
43. Wijeyeratne YD, Joshi R, Heptinstall S. Ticagrelor, a P2Y$_{12}$ antagonist for use in acute coronary syndromes. Expert Rev Clin Cardiol. 2012;5:257–69.
44. van Giezen JJ, Nilsson L, Berntsson P, Wissing BM, Giordanetto F, Tomlinson W, Greasley PJ. Ticagrelor binds to human P2Y(12) independently from ADP but antagonizes ADP-induced receptor signaling and platelet aggregation. J Thromb Haemost. 2009;7: 1556–65.

45. Teng R, Oliver S, Hayes MA, Butler K. Absorption, distribution, metabolism, and excretion of ticagrelor in healthy subjects. Drug Metab Dispos. 2010;38(9):1514–21.

46. Husted S, Emanuelsson H, Heptinstall S, Sandset PM, Wickens M, Peters G. Pharmacodynamics, pharmacokinetics, and safety of the oral reversible P2Y12 antagonist AZD6140 with aspirin in patients with atherosclerosis: a double-blind comparison to clopidogrel with aspirin. Eur Heart J. 2006;27:1038–47.

47. Storey RF, Husted S, Harrington RA, Heptinstall S, Wilcox RG, Peters G, Wickens M, Emanuelsson H, Gurbel P, Grande P, Cannon CP. Inhibition of platelet aggregation by AZD6140, a reversible oral P2Y12 receptor antagonist, compared with clopidogrel in patients with acute coronary syndromes. J Am Coll Cardiol. 2007;50:1852–6.

48. Gurbel PA, Bliden KP, Butler K, Tantry US, Gesheff T, Wei C, Teng R, Antonino MJ, Patil SB, Karunakaran A, Kereiakes DJ, Parris C, Purdy D, Wilson V, Ledley GS, Storey RF. Randomized double-blind assessment of the ONSET and OFFSET of the antiplatelet effects of ticagrelor versus clopidogrel in patients with stable coronary artery disease: the ONSET/OFFSET study. Circulation. 2009;120:2577–85.

49. Gurbel PA, Bliden KP, Butler K, Antonino MJ, Wei C, Teng R, Rasmussen L, Storey RF, Nielsen T, Eikelboom JW, Sabe-Affaki G, Husted S, Kereiakes DJ, Henderson D, Patel DV, Tantry US. Response to ticagrelor in clopidogrel nonresponders and responders and effect of switching therapies: the RESPOND study. Circulation. 2010;121:1188–99.

50. Storey RF, Angiolillo DJ, Patil SB, Desai B, Ecob R, Husted S, Emanuelsson H, Cannon CP, Becker RC, Wallentin L. Inhibitory effects of ticagrelor compared with clopidogrel on platelet function in patients with acute coronary syndromes: the PLATO (PLATelet inhibition and patient Outcomes) PLATELET substudy. J Am Coll Cardiol. 2010;56:1456–62.

51. James S, Akerblom A, Cannon CP, Emanuelsson H, Husted S, Katus H, Skene A, Steg PG, Storey RF, Harrington R, Becker R, Wallentin L. Comparison of ticagrelor, the first reversible oral P2Y(12) receptor antagonist, with clopidogrel in patients with acute coronary syndromes: rationale, design, and baseline characteristics of the PLATelet inhibition and patient outcomes (PLATO) trial. Am Heart J. 2009;157:599–605.

52. Wallentin L, Becker RC, Budaj A, Cannon CP, Emanuelsson H, Held C, Horrow J, Husted S, James S, Katus H, Mahaffey KW,

Scirica BM, Skene A, Steg PG, Storey RF, Harrington RA, Freij A, Thorsén M, PLATO Investigators. Ticagrelor versus clopidogrel in patients with acute coronary syndromes. N Engl J Med. 2009;361:1045–57.

53. Iyú D, Glenn JR, White AE, Fox SC, van Giezen H, Nylander S, Heptinstall S. Mode of action of P2Y12 antagonists as inhibitors of platelet function. Thromb Haemost. 2010;105:96–106.

54. Storey RF, Becker RC, Harrington RA, Husted S, James SK, Cools F, Steg PG, Khurmi NS, Emanuelsson H, Cooper A, Cairns R, Cannon CP, Wallentin L. Characterization of dyspnoea in PLATO study patients treated with ticagrelor or clopidogrel and its association with clinical outcomes. Eur Heart J. 2011;32:2945–53.

55. van Giezen JJ, Sidaway J, Glaves P, Kirk I, Björkman JA. Ticagrelor inhibits adenosine uptake in vitro and enhances adenosine-mediated hyperemia responses in a canine model. J Cardiovasc Pharmacol Ther. 2012;17:164–72.

56. Iyú D, Glenn JR, White AE, Fox SC, Heptinstall S. Adenosine derived from ADP can contribute to inhibition of platelet aggregation in the presence of a P2Y12 antagonist. Arterioscler Thromb Vasc Biol. 2011;31:416–22.

57. Mahaffey KW, Wojdyla DM, Carroll K, Becker RC, Storey RF, Angiolillo DJ, Held C, Cannon CP, James S, Pieper KS, Horrow J, Harrington RA, Wallentin L. Ticagrelor compared with clopidogrel by geographic region in the platelet inhibition and patient outcomes (PLATO) trial. Circulation. 2011;124:544–54.

58. Fox SC, Behan MWH, Heptinstall S. Inhibition of ADP-induced intracellular Ca2+ responses and platelet aggregation by the P2Y12 receptor antagonists AR-C69931MX and clopidogrel is enhanced by prostaglandin E1. Cell Calcium. 2004;35:39–46.

59. Cattaneo M, Lecchi A. Inhibition of the platelet $P2Y_{12}$ receptor for adenosine diphosphate potentiates the antiplatelet effect of prostacyclin. J Thromb Haemost. 2007;5:577–82.

60. Iyú D, Glenn JR, White AE, Fox SC, Dovlatova N, Heptinstall S. P2Y(12) and EP3 antagonists promote the inhibitory effects of natural modulators of platelet aggregation that act via cAMP. Platelets. 2011;22:504–15.

61. FDA. Advisory Committee Briefing Document. Ticagrelor. 2010. http://www.fda.gov/downloads/AdvisoryCommitteesMeetingMaterials/Drugs/CardiovascularandRenalDrugsAdvisoryCommittee/UCM220197.pdf Accessed 1 Jan 2012.

62. FDA. News release. FDA approves blood-thinning drug Brilinta to treat acute coronary syndromes. 2011. http://www.fda.gov/

NewsEvents/Newsroom/PressAnnouncements/ucm263964.htm
Accessed 1 Jan 2012.

63. Srinivasan S, Mir F, Huang JS, Khasawneh FT, Lam SC, Le
Breton GC. The P2Y12 antagonists, 2-methylthioadenosine
5'-monophosphate triethyammonium salt and cangrelor
(ARC69931MX), can inhibit human platelet aggregation through
a Gi-independent increase in cAMP levels. J Biol Chem.
2009;284:16108–17.

64. Storey RF, Oldroyd KG, Wilcox RG. Open multicentre study of
the P2T receptor antagonist AR-C69931MX assessing safety,
tolerability and activity in patients with acute coronary syndromes. Thromb Haemost. 2001;85:401–7.

65. Angiolillo DJ, Firstenberg MS, Price MJ, Tummala PE, Hutyra
M, Welsby IJ, Voeltz MD, Chandna H, Ramaiah C, Brtko M,
Cannon L, Dyke C, Liu T, Montalescot G, Manoukian SV, Prats
J, Topol EJ, for the BRIDGE Investigators. Bridging antiplatelet
therapy with cangrelor in patients undergoing cardiac surgery. A
randomized controlled trial. J Am Med Assoc. 2012;307
(3):265–74.

66. Steinhubl SR, Oh JJ, Oestreich JH, Ferraris S, Charnigo R, Akers
WS. Transitioning patients from cangrelor to clopidogrel: pharmacodynamic evidence of a competitive effect. Thromb Res.
2008;121:527–34.

67. Dovlatova NL, Jakubowski JA, Sugidachi A, Heptinstall S. The
reversible P2Y antagonist cangrelor influences the ability of the
active metabolites of clopidogrel and prasugrel to produce irreversible inhibition of platelet function. J Thromb Haemost.
2008;6:1153–9.

68. Ueno M, Rao SV, Angiolillo DJ. Elinogrel: pharmacological
principles, preclinical and early phase clinical testing. Future
Cardiol. 2010;6:445–53.

69. Bult H, Fret HR, Jordaens FH, Herman AG. Dipyridamole
potentiates platelet inhibition by nitric oxide. Thromb Haemost.
1991;66:343–9.

70. Dawicki DD, Agarwal KC, Parks Jr RE. Role of adenosine
uptake and metabolism by blood cells in the antiplatelet actions
of dipyridamole, dilazep and nitrobenzylthioinosine. Biochem
Pharmacol. 1985;34:3965–72.

71. Diener HC, Cunha L, Forbes C, Sivenius J, Smets P, Lowenthal
A. European stroke prevention study. 2. Dipyridamole and ace-
tylsalicylic acid in the secondary prevention of stroke. J Neurol
Sci. 1996;143:1–13.

72. Liu Y, Shakur Y, Yoshitake M, Kambayashi JiJ. Cilostazol (pletal): a dual inhibitor of cyclic nucleotide phosphodiesterase type 3 and adenosine uptake. Cardiovasc Drug Rev. 2001;19:369–86.
73. Hagemeyer CE, Peter K. Targeting the platelet integrin GPIIb/IIIa. Curr Pharm Des. 2010;16:4119–33.
74. Zhao L, Bath PM, Fox S, May J, Judge H, Lösche W, Heptinstall S. The effects of GPIIb-IIIa antagonists and a combination of three other antiplatelet agents on platelet-leukocyte interactions. Curr Med Res Opin. 2003;19:178–86.
75. Zhao L, Bath PM, May J, Lösche W, Heptinstall S. P-selectin, tissue factor and CD40 ligand expression on platelet-leucocyte conjugates in the presence of a GPIIb/IIIa antagonist. Platelets. 2003;14:473–80.
76. Tricoci P, Huang Z, Held C, Moliterno DJ, Armstrong PW, Van de Werf F, White HD, Aylward PE, Wallentin L, Chen E, Lokhnygina Y, Pei J, Leonardi S, Rorick TL, Kilian AM, Jennings LH, Ambrosio G, Bode C, Cequier A, Cornel JH, Diaz R, Erkan A, Huber K, Hudson MP, Jiang L, Jukema JW, Lewis BS, Lincoff AM, Montalescot G, Nicolau JC, Ogawa H, Pfisterer M, Prieto JC, Ruzyllo W, Sinnaeve PR, Storey RF, Valgimigli M, Whellan DJ, Widimsky P, Strony J, Harrington RA, Mahaffey KW, TRACER Investigators. Thrombin-receptor antagonist vorapaxar in acute coronary syndromes. N Engl J Med. 2012;366: 20–33.
77. Ungerer M, Rosport K, Bültmann A, Piechatzek R, Uhland K, Schlieper P, Gawaz M, Münch G. Novel antiplatelet drug revacept (dimeric glycoprotein VI-Fc) specifically and efficiently inhibited collagen-induced platelet aggregation without affecting general hemostasis in humans. Circulation. 2011;123:1891–9.
78. Firbas C, Siller-Matula JM, Jilma B. Targeting von willebrand factor and platelet glycoprotein Ib receptor. Expert Rev Cardiovasc Ther. 2010;8:1689–701.
79. Heptinstall S, Espinosa DI, Manolopoulos P, Glenn JR, White AE, Johnson A, Dovlatova N, Fox SC, May JA, Hermann D, Magnusson O, Stefansson K, Hartman D, Gurney M. DG-041 inhibits the EP3 prostanoid receptor--a new target for inhibition of platelet function in atherothrombotic disease. Platelets. 2008;19:605–13.
80. Singh J, Zeller W, Zhou N, Hategen G, Mishra R, Polozov A, Yu P, Onua E, Zhang J, Zembower D, Kiselyov A, Ramírez JL, Sigthorsson G, Bjornsson JM, Thorsteinsdottir M, Andrésson T, Bjarnadottir M, Magnusson O, Fabre JE, Stefansson K, Gurney

ME. Antagonists of the EP3 receptor for prostaglandin E2 are novel antiplatelet agents that do not prolong bleeding. ACS Chem Biol. 2009;4:115–26.

81. Fox SC, May JA, Johnson A, Hermann D, Streiter D, Hartman D, Heptinstall S, Effects on platelet function of an EP3 receptor antagonist used alone and in combination with a $P2Y_{12}$ antagonist both *in-vitro* and *ex-vivo* in human volunteers. Platelets 2012.

Chapter 2
Antiplatelet Drug Resistance and Variability in Response: The Role of Antiplatelet Therapy Monitoring

Paul A. Gurbel and Udaya S. Tantry

Introduction

Atherothrombotic complications are the primary causes of cardiovascular mortality and morbidity and antiplatelet therapy constitutes the mainstay of initial and long-term pharmacologic treatment to prevent atherothrombotic events [1]. The common underlying pathological basis for the development of atherothrombotic events is occlusive platelet rich thrombus generation at the site of plaque rupture. The subendothelial matrix with collagen and von Willebrand factor (vWF) is

P.A. Gurbel, M.D. (✉)
Sinai Center for Thrombosis Research,
Sinai Hospital of Baltimore,
2401 W. Belvedere Ave, Baltimore, MD 21215, USA
e-mail: pgurbel@lifebridgehealth.org

Johns Hopkins University School of Medicine,
Baltimore, MD, USA

U.S. Tantry, Ph.D.
Sinai Center for Thrombosis Research,
Sinai Hospital of Baltimore,
2401 W. Belvedere Ave, Baltimore, MD 21215, USA
e-mail: utantry@lifebridgehealth.org

A. Ferro, D.A. Garcia (eds.), *Antiplatelet and Anticoagulation* 45
Therapy, Current Cardiovascular Therapy,
DOI 10.1007/978-1-4471-4297-3_2,
© Springer-Verlag London 2013

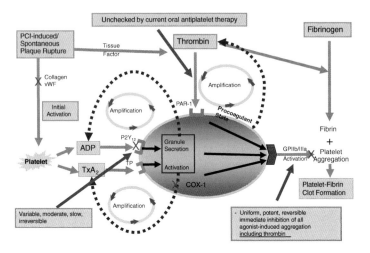

FIGURE 2.1 Mechanisms of platelet activation and inhibition

exposed after vascular injury and platelet adhesion is pro-
moted. Platelets are activated following the binding of collagen
and vWF to specific membrane receptors. Thrombin generated by exposed tissue factor is also a major platelet agonist.
Platelet activation results in the release of adenosine diphosphate from dense granules and thromboxane A_2 generated
by the cyclooxygenase-1 (COX-1) pathway. COX-1 converts
arachidonic acid (originating from membrane phospholipids)
to prostaglandin $(PG)H_2$ and platelet specific thromboxane
(Tx) synthase converts PGH_2 to $Tx A_2$. By autocrine and
paracrine mechanisms, these agonists are responsible for the
amplification of platelet activation. Although TxA_2 and ADP
act synergistically during platelet aggregation, continuous
ADP-$P2Y_{12}$ receptor signaling is essential for the sustained
activation of the GPIIb/IIIa receptor and stable thrombus
generation. Platelet activation exposes the phosphotidyl serine surface providing binding sites for coagulation factors and
the generation of thrombin. The fibrin network generated by
thrombin activity binds to the aggregated platelets and forms
stable clot at the site of vascular injury (Fig. 2.1) [1].
    Occlusive thrombus generation is also responsible for
microembolization that results in microvascular dysfunction
following stroke and myocardial infarction. Platelets are not

only central to these thrombotic processes ("platelet hypothesis") but also play important roles in atherosclerosis, coagulation and inflammation [2]. Platelet activation is a complex process involving many receptors and signaling pathways. Therefore, more effective prevention of thrombotic events in high risk patients has been observed with a strategy of inhibition of multiple pathways [2]. Aspirin inhibits the cyclooxygenase-1 enzyme, $P2Y_{12}$ receptor blockers inhibit the ability of ADP to activate platelets and reversible glycoprotein (GP) IIb/IIIa receptor blockers inhibit activated platelets from binding to the dimeric fibrinogen molecule (Fig. 2.1). GP IIb/IIIa receptor inhibitors are used in addition to dual antiplatelet therapy of aspirin and $P2Y_{12}$ receptor blocker (DAPT) during the highest risk clinical settings [1, 3]. The determination of optimal platelet inhibition is dependent on the degree of ischemic risk, and is counterbalanced by the risk of bleeding. Optimization of antiplatelet therapy to prevent ischemic event occurrences without increasing excessive bleeding is of great clinical importance [3].

Clinical efficacy of dual antiplatelet therapy has been demonstrated in large scale clinical trials. In these clinical trials, a non-selective "one size fits all" approach has been implemented without evaluating the platelet response in the individual patient. However, ex vivo laboratory evaluation of individual antiplatelet response in translation research studies indicated a wide response variability where a desired antiplatelet response was not observed with the prescribed dosing regimens in a substantial percentage of patients. This phenomenon was described as "antiplatelet resistance or nonresponsiveness" [4]. Moreover, continued occurrence of recurrent ischemic events among selected patients with high on treatment platelet reactivity or among patients exhibiting antiplatelet resistance again highlighted the importance of limitations of uniform dual antiplatelet treatment strategy. On the other hand, excessively low platelet reactivity observed in some patients on clopidogrel therapy and especially in those on prasugrel or ticagrelor therapy may be associated with unnecessary increased risk of bleeding. Thus, the central role of platelets in the genesis of thrombosis and bleeding and the high treatment failure rate (~10–12 %) observed in major clinical trials of DAPT are 3 major reasons for platelet function testing in patients at high risk of cardiovascular disease. By monitoring platelet function during antiplatelet therapy, one may be able to ensure that an acceptable level of on-treatment platelet reactivity is present [5].

Response Variability and Resistance to Antiplatelet Drugs

The phenomenon of antiplatelet drug "resistance" may be due to a (a) **pharmacokinetic** mechanism where a reduced absorption or conversion to an active metabolite leads to inadequate availability of drug/active metabolite to sufficiently block the respective receptor pathways; (b) **pharmacodynamic** mechanism where decreased response of platelets to the drug occurs due to variability in platelet response secondary to increased turnover of platelets, increased responsiveness of platelets to certain agonist, genetic variability of receptors or intracellular signaling mechanism, or interactions with other drugs at the active site of the receptors; or (c) **treatment failure** where patients may suffer recurrent vascular events despite inhibition of the platelet activation pathways by antiplatelet therapy [4].

Multiple signaling pathways mediate platelet activation and are responsible for the occurrence of thrombotic events. Thus a treatment strategy directed against a single pathway cannot be expected to prevent the occurrence of all ischemic events and treatment failure following single antiplatelet strategy alone is not sufficient evidence of drug resistance. "Resistance" or nonresponsiveness to an antiplatelet is provided by persistent activity of the specific target of the antiplatelet agent. Since the active metabolite of clopidogrel irreversibly inhibits the $P2Y_{12}$ receptor, evidence for nonresponsiveness to clopidogrel is provided by high on-treatment $P2Y_{12}$ reactivity. For aspirin, the identification of resistance would use a laboratory technique that detects residual activity of the COX-1 enzyme. So called "resistance" to antiplatelet drugs is more meaningful only when the biochemical phenomenon of resistance is measured by a well-established laboratory method that has a strong relation to the occurrence of adverse clinical outcomes. Moreover, it will be clinically more useful when the increased risk can be effectively overcome by alternative therapies or more potent antiplatelet drugs without an excessively increased bleeding risk [4].

Aspirin

Aspirin

Aspirin is the bedrock of antiplatelet therapy in coronary artery disease patients [1, 3]. A loading dose of 300–325 mg is recommended during acute settings of ACS and PCI whereas 75–162 mg is recommended for long-term, and most often, life-long therapy. Similar clinical efficacy was associated with daily aspirin doses between 75 and 1,500 mg in a meta-analysis. However, there was a 50 % reduction in efficacy with doses <75 mg [6]. Similarly, no significant differences in the 30 day outcome of cardiovascular death, MI or stroke and no differences in major bleeding were observed between 75–100 mg and 300–325 mg daily aspirin doses in the Double-dose versus standard-dose clopidogrel and high-dose versus low-dose aspirin in individuals undergoing percutaneous coronary intervention for acute coronary syndromes (CURRENT OASIS)-7 trial that included ACS patients undergoing PCI [7].

Aspirin is readily absorbed in the upper gastrointestinal tract. Peak plasma levels of aspirin are observed within 40 min and platelet inhibition and also prolongation of bleeding time can be observed within an hour. Aspirin is mainly metabolized by intestinal and liver human carboxyesterase (HCE)-2 to acetyl and salicylate moieties [1]. Aspirin has a half-life of 15–20 min whereas salicylate has a half life of 3–6 h. Platelet inhibition has been observed even before the appearance of aspirin in the systemic circulation suggesting that acetylation of the platelet cyclooxygenase (COX)-1 takes place in the prehepatic circulation [1]. Thromboxane metabolite measurement in serum or thromboxane-dependent platelet function measurements are considered surrogate measures of aspirin bioavailability in preference to salicylate levels in the venous blood [8].

Antiplatelet Effects of Aspirin

The antiplatelet effect of aspirin has been attributed primarily to irreversible acetylation of a serine residue (Ser529) in COX-1 present in platelets. Aspirin prevents access of arachidonic acid (AA) to the catalytic site (Tyr 385) of COX-1 and thereby inhibits the synthesis of PGH_2. Subsequently, generation of TxA_2 and TxA_2-induced platelet aggregation are inhibited for the lifespan of the platelet. TxA_2 is highly unstable in aqueous solution and is rapidly hydrolyzed to the stable physiologically inactive metabolite, TxB_2 [9]. Aspirin also acetylates serine 516 of the COX-2 enzyme and inhibits COX-2 mediated prostonoid synthesis, however, acetylated COX-2 is capable of converting AA into 15R-hydroxyeicosatetraenoic acid (15 R-HETE). The 15R-HETE can be converted by 5-lipooxygenase into 15-epi-lipoxin A4 which can stimulate nitric oxide release to inhibit leukocyte-endothelial interaction. The latter anti-inflammatory property can be attributed to aspirin [10]. Aspirin rapidly acetylates the COX-1 enzyme 166 times more effectively than COX-2. Aspirin only inhibits COX-1 activity and not thromboxane synthase activity. It has been demonstrated that even residual 10 % capacity to generate thromboxane *in vivo* is sufficient to generate thromboxane–dependent platelet activation [11]. Furthermore, more than 95 % inhibition of thromboxane synthesis is believed necessary to observe clinical efficacy from aspirin treatment [12]. Even low levels of COX-2 expression in platelets may induce platelet aggregation in the presence of aspirin [8]. In addition, endothelial cells and monocytes/macrophages can rapidly (2–4 h) recover from the aspirin effect by resynthesizing the COX-2 enzyme and may contribute PGH_2 to platelets that synthesize TxA_2 by thromboxane synthase (transcellular TxA_2 synthesis) [13]. This phenomenon may be important at the site of plaque rupture where monocytes and macrophages coexist with platelets during thrombosis development and may overcome the antithombotic effect of aspirin [14]. Moreover, in patients with vascular inflammation, the same extra platelet sources of TxA_2 may affect the protective clinical effect of aspirin therapy. Urinary 11-dehydro-TxB_2 (11-dh TxB_2) levels reflect cumulative *in vivo* production of TxA_2. In addition to suggesting an insufficient antiplatelet effect, elevated urinary 11-dehydroTxB_2 levels may also indicate residual COX-2 activity in inflammatory cells. Although in normal conditions COX-2 comprises less than 10 % of COX present in platelets, under conditions of high platelet turnover such as post-coronary artery bypass surgery, its expression may be as high as 60 % and may contribute to high levels of TxA_2 production despite COX-1 inhibition induced by low dose aspirin (75–81 mg/day) therapy (Fig. 2.2)[14, 15].

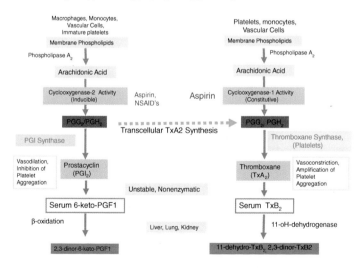

FIGURE 2.2 Mechanism of action of aspirin

Aspirin Resistance

A reliable and specific laboratory method to identify aspirin resistance has not yet been uniformly accepted by investigators. It is important to note that shear as well as stimulation by ADP, collagen and epinephrine can activate platelets in the presence of complete COX-1 blockade. Laboratory methods, including point-of-care methods that use the latter agonists to stimulate platelets, do not solely indicate the level of COX-1 activity and are considered "COX-1 nonspecific methods" [8, 16].

The optimal definition of resistance or non-responsiveness to aspirin is the demonstration of residual activity of the primary target of aspirin, namely the COX-1 enzyme. Measurement of serum TxB_2 or agonist-induced TxB_2 in platelet rich plasma and AA-induced platelet aggregation are the most specific assays to indicate COX-1 activity ("COX-1 specific methods"). However, serum TxB_2 measurement may be affected by non-platelet sources such as leukocytes. The VerifyNow aspirin assay measures AA- induced agglutination of platelets to fibrinogen coated beads in whole blood; the thrombelastography (TEG) Platelet Mapping assay measures AA-induced platelet-fibrin clot strength in whole blood; and the Multiplate analyzer is an impedance aggregometer that employs AA as an agonist in whole blood. Urinary 11-dehydro (dH) TxB_2 excretion measurements have been used to indicate COX-1 activity and aspirin responsiveness [8]. However, 11-dH-TxB_2 represents whole body TxA_2 production and may also be influenced by non-platelet sources especially in pathological conditions of inflammation and high-risk cardiovascular disease (see above) (Fig. 2.3) [8]. Finally, the least specific indicator of COX-1 activity may be the Platelet Function Analyzer (PFA)-100 assay that employs stimulation with collagen and epinephrine in the presence of shear. In addition to vWF levels, the closure time measurement in PFA-100 is also dependent on ABO blood group, leukocyte count and mean platelet count [17].

A systematic review of various studies revealed that after adjusting for differences in definition, dosage, and population, the prevalence of aspirin resistance was dependent on dosage and laboratory methods. A >300 mg/day dosage was

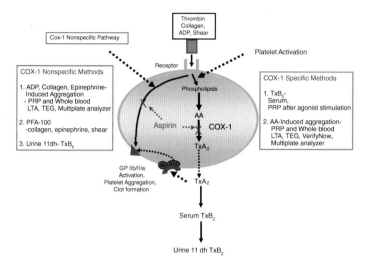

FIGURE 2.3 Laboratory evaluation of aspirin responsiveness

associated with a significantly lower prevalence of resistance compared to a <100 mg/day dosage (19 % vs. 26 % respectively, $p < 0.001$). A lower unadjusted prevalence of resistance (6 %) was observed with arachidonic acid-induced aggregation measured by light transmittance aggregometry (LTA) compared to a 26 % prevalence with the PFA-100 method [18]. Based on the different *ex-vivo* methods and criteria used to define aspirin resistance, it is not surprising that there is wide variability in the reported occurrence of aspirin resistance (<1–57 %) (Tables 2.1 and 2.2) [19–42].

Aspirin Resistance Demonstrated in Pharmacodynamic Studies

Platelet aspirin resistance was found to be uncommon in compliant percutaneous coronary intervention (PCI) patients treated with high dose aspirin (325 mg per day) when measured by COX-1 specific assays such as AA-induced light transmittance aggregometry LTA and TEG [30]. In another study of patients with a history of myocardial infarction, 9 % of patients

TABLE 2.1 Studies demonstrating aspirin resistance

Investigators	n		ASA dose (mg/day)	Time	Method	Criteria for aspirin resistance (AR)	% AR
Hurlen et al. [19]	143	AMI	75–160	2–24 h	PAR	PAR <0.82	9.8
						PAR <0.82 after additional ASA	1.4
Buchanan et al. [20]	40	CABG	325		Bleeding time platelet TxA$_2$, 12-HETE and platelet adhesion	No prolongation of bleeding time above baseline	43
Buchanan et al. [21]	287	CABG	325	24 h 2 years follow-up	Bleeding time	No prolongation of bleeding time above baseline	54.7
Grotemeyer et al. [22]	180	Stroke	1,500	1 year follow-up	PR	Normal PR index (>1.25) at 2 or 12 h	33.3

Study	N	Population	ASA dose	Follow-up	Test	Definition	%
Gum et al. [23, 24]	325	Stable CAD	325	≥7 days	LTA- AA and ADP	>70 % ADP induced aggregation+AA (0.5 mg/ml) induced >20 % after ASA	5.5
				2 years follow-up	PFA- 100 collagen/ADP or collagen/ EPI	Normal (<193 s) collagen/EPI closure time after ASA	9.5
Eikelboom et al. [25] (HOPE Study)	976	CVD	75–325	5 years follow-up	Urinary 11-dehydro TxA$_2$ at baseline	Elevated urinary 11-dehydro TxB$_2$ - upper quartile - 33.7 ng/mmol creatinine	25
Eikelboom et al [26] (CHARISMA Study)	3,261	High-risk ATH pts	75–162	median 28 months	Urinary 11-dH-TxB2 after 1 month of randomization	Elevated urinary 11-dehydro TxB$_2$ - upper quartile- Median 72.7 ng/ mmol creatinine	25
Wang et al. [27]	422	Stable CAD	81–325	≥7 days	RPFA	ARU>550	23

(continued)

TABLE 2.1 (continued)

Investigators	n	ASA dose (mg/day)	Time	Method	Criteria for aspirin resistance (AR)	% AR
Chen et al. [28]	151	Non-urgent PCI	81–325	≥7 days	RPFA CK-MB+TnI	ARU>550	19.2
Gonzalez-Conejero et al. [29]	24	HS	100 and 500	2 weeks	PA – 1 mM AA or 10 μg/ml Collagen, 11-dehydro TxA$_2$ PFA-100, genotyping.	<300 s closer time	33.3 (100 mg) 0 (500 mg)
Tantry et al. [30]	223	PCI	325	Long-term	LTA -1 mM AA	>20 % aggregation	<1.0
					TEG- 1 mM AA	>50 %	<1.0

PAR platelet aggregation ratio, *AMI* acute myocardial infarction, *ASA* aspirin, *CABG* coronary artery bypass surgery grafting, *HETE* hydroxyeicosatetraenoic acid, *PVD* peripheral vascular disease, *TxA$_2$* thromboxane A$_2$, *HOPE* heart outcomes prevention evaluation, *PR* platelet reactivity, *CAD* coronary artery disease, *ADP* adenosine diphosphate, *11-dH-TxB2* 11-dehydro- thromboxane B$_2$, *MI* myocardial infarction, *CHARISMA* clopidogrel for high atherothrombotic risk and ischemic stabilization, management and avoidance, *LTA* light transmittance aggregometry, *TEG* thrombelastography, *PCI* percutaneous coronary intervention, *HS* healthy subjects, *COLL/EPI* collagen/epinephrine, *ASA* aspirin, *ATH* atherosclerosis, *PFA* platelet function analyzer, *ARu* aspirin resistance units, *RPFA* rapid platelet function analyzer, *HS* healthy subjects

TABLE 2.2 Clinical relevance of aspirin resistance

Investigators	n	Method	Clinical outcome
Muller [47]	100 PVD	Whole blood aggregometry	87 % increase in incidence of reocclusion
Grotmeyer et al. [22]	180 Post-stroke	Platelet aggregates	10x increase in vascular events
Eikelboom et al. [25]	976 HOPE trial	Urinary 11-dH- TxB_2	1.8x increase in MI/stroke/death risk in upper quartile
Eikelboom et al. [26]	3,261 CHARISMA trial	Urinary 11-dH- TxB_2	1.66x increase in MI/stroke/death risk in upper quartile
Gum et al. [23]	325 Stable CAD	LTA	3.12x increase in MI/stroke/death
Tantry et al. [4]	223 Elective	LTA and TEG-2 mm AA	Aspirin resistance = 0.4 %, 1 patient-stent thrombosis
Chen et al. [28]	151 Elective	LTA and TEG-2 mm AA	2.9X increase in myonecrosis
Lev et al. [37]	150 PCI	LTA –1.6 mM AA RPFA-(propyl gallate)	Elevated CK-MB
Marcucci et al. [38]	146 MI/PCI	PFA-100 (Coll/EPI)	↑ 1 Year MACE
Gianetti et al. [39]	175 (SA/AMI)	PFA-100 (Coll-EPI and ADP)	6 months outcome-HR = 8.5-
Foussas et al. [40]	612 (SA/UA)	PFA-100 (Coll-EPI)	1 year CV death and rehosp-HR = 2.7

(continued)

TABLE 2.2 (continued)

Investigators	n	Method	Clinical outcome
Malek et al. [41]	91 (PCI)	PFA-100 (Coll-EPI and ADP)	Unfavorable in-hospital outcome
Borna et al. [42]	135 (ACS)	PFA-100 (Coll-EPI and ADP)	ASA-R associated with STEMI
Snoep et al. [49]	1,813 pts with events	Various methods	3.8x (pooled odds ratio) increase in all cardiovascular outcomes
Cresente et al. [50]	3,003 pts	PFA-100 (collagen-EPI)	2.35x increase in vascular events
Reny et al. [51]	2,693 metaanalysis	PFA-100 (coll-EPI)	2.1x increase in recurrent ischemic events

PVD peripheral vascular disease, *HOPE* heart outcomes prevention Evaluation, *11-dH-TxB2* 11-dehydro- thromboxane B₂, *MI* myocardial infarction, *CHARISMA* clopidogrel for high atherothrombotic risk and ischemic stabilization, management and avoidance, *LTA* light transmittance aggregometry, *TEG* thrombelastography, *PCI* percutaneous coronary intervention, *CK-MB* creatinine-MB, *COLL/EPI* collagen/epinephrine, *ADP* adenosine diphosphate, *ASA* aspirin, *SA/UA* stable angina/ unstable angina, *ACS* acute coronary syndrome, *STEMI* St-segment elevation myocardial infarction, *PFA* platelet function analyzer

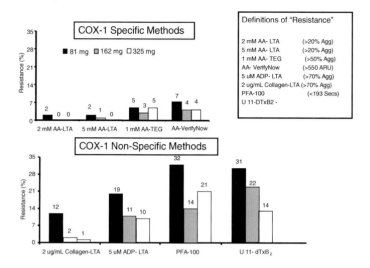

FIGURE 2.4 Prevalence of aspirin resistance (Adapted from Gurbel et al. [32])

were found to be noncompliant with aspirin therapy and only one patient was resistant to 325 mg aspirin therapy as measured by AA-induced LTA [31]. In a prospective, randomized, double-blind, double crossover investigation studying the effect of aspirin dosing (81, 162, 325 mg daily) on platelet function in patients with stable coronary artery disease (n = 120) measured by multiple assays, it was found that aspirin non-responsiveness was rare (1–6 %) using methods that employed arachidonic acid stimulation (LTA, VerifyNow Aspirin assay, TEG) at all doses of aspirin. When other agonists were used, the prevalence of resistance was 1–27 %. The prevalence was 23 % based on the measurement of urinary 11-dh TxB_2 excretion [32]. Moreover, a dose dependent response to aspirin treatment was observed when collagen, ADP, and shear were used to activate platelets. The latter occurred in the presence of near complete inhibition of the COX-1 enzyme activity as measured by arachidonic acid-induced platelet aggregation, indicating that aspirin may have non-COX-1 mediated dose dependent effects in platelets (Fig. 2.4) [32].

In a *post hoc* analysis of the Aspirin-Induced Platelet Effect (ASPECT) study, greater platelet reactivity and a higher prevalence of aspirin resistance were present in patients with diabetes compared to patients without diabetes. Aspirin doses of >81 mg daily (162–325 mg) were associated with similar rates of resistance and platelet function in patients with and without diabetes. It was hypothesized, therefore, that a higher aspirin dosing strategy than 81 mg QD in patients with diabetes may be associated with enhanced platelet inhibition and better protection against athero-thrombotic event occurrence [43]. Various mechanisms have been proposed to explain the attenuated antiplatelet effect of aspirin therapy in diabetes, such as reduced drug bioavail-ability, accelerated platelet turnover, and glycosylation of platelet membrane proteins [44]. The presence of COX-2 in immature platelets may contribute to aspirin-insensitive TxA_2 generation, as can the presence of COX-2 in leukocytes that participate in transcellular thromboxane A2 synthesis (see above) [8]. Lower platelet reactivity was demonstrated in patients with diabetes treated with twice-daily dosing com-pared to once-daily dosing [45, 46]. In addition, a dose-dependent effect on serum TxB_2 levels has been reported irrespective of the frequency of dosing that did not correlate with platelet function measurements, most notably aggregation stimulated by arachidonic acid [46]. Moreover, these results demon-strated that additional antiplatelet effects weren't achieved by increasing the aspirin dose to >162 mg daily suggesting that 162 mg daily aspirin may be the optimal dose in patients with CAD and diabetes [47].

Clinical Relevance of Aspirin Resistance

Numerous studies using different assays to measure aspirin responsiveness demonstrated that aspirin resistance is associ-ated with worse clinical outcomes (Table 2.2) [22, 24, 28–32, 38–42, 48–51]. In a systematic review and meta-analysis of various studies linking aspirin resistance to clinical outcomes utilizing different methods, an odds ratio of all cardiovascular outcomes of 3.8 (95 %CI; 2.3–6.1) for aspirin resistance was observed [49]. Multiple studies have correlated the occurrence of adverse clinical outcomes with aspirin resistance measured by the PFA-100. In another systematic review of 53 studies comprising 6,450 patients, a prevalence of 27 % aspirin resistance with a 1.63 relative risk (95 % CI; 1.16–2.28) for vascular events was demonstrated [50]. Similarly, in another meta-analysis of prospective studies, aspirin resistance as measured by the PFA-100 was associated with recurrent ischemic events with an OR of 2.1 (95 % CI; 1.4–3.4, $p < 0.001$) [51]. Urinary 11-dh-TxB$_2$ excretion has been used as an indicator of aspirin responsiveness and also has been identified as an indicator of ischemic risk in clinical studies [25, 26].

Thus, taken together, all of these studies indicate that noncompliance, various assessment methods, and underdosing may all be important factors responsible for the reported variability in laboratory aspirin resistance estimates. It has also been demonstrated that aspirin resistance may be associated with clopidogrel resistance [37, 52]. Moreover, aspirin resistant patients have been shown to exhibit high platelet reactivity to various agonists such as collagen and ADP in addition to arachidonic acid [53]. Therefore, aspirin resistance as measured in these studies may mark a platelet reactivity phenotype indicative of high risk for ischemic events. To date, no convincing data are available regarding the utility of measuring platelet response to multiple agonists in stratifying the risk for ischemic events. High platelet reactivity to multiple agonists may not be due to independent responses but rather indicate a global high platelet reactivity phenotype [53].

Concomitant use of other nonsteroidal anti-inflammatory drugs may diminish aspirin's antiplatelet effect and influence aspirin responsiveness [1]. By reversibly binding to platelet COX-1, specific NSAIDs limit the access of aspirin to its binding site [54]. It has been reported that concomitant use of aspirin with NSAIDs may be associated with an increased risk of CV events [55, 56]. Recently, co-administration of ranitidine, a histamine (H$_2$) receptor antagonist often prescribed along with aspirin to reduce gastrointestinal side effects, with aspirin (325 mg/day) was associated with poorer inhibition of platelet aggregation induced by AA, collagen, and ADP in healthy volunteers compared to aspirin therapy alone [57].

The relation between gene polymorphisms and aspirin responsiveness is unclear. Various studies have suggested the influence of genetic polymorphisms of COX-1, COX-2, GPIIIa, $P2Y_{12}$ and $P2Y_1$ on aspirin responsiveness. A recent systematic review of 31 studies involving 50 polymorphisms in 11 genes in 2,834 subjects revealed that only the PlA1/A2 polymorphism in the GPIIIa receptor was significantly associated with aspirin resistance in healthy subjects (OR 2.36, 95 % CI: 1.24–4.49, p=0.009). However, the effect was diminished in patients with cardiovascular disease [58].

In addition to the mechanisms described above to explain aspirin resistance, other factors that are known to augment platelet reactivity such as smoking, diabetes, hyperlipidemia, may affect the prevalence of aspirin resistance and hence the occurrence of adverse clinical outcomes in patients treated with aspirin. Measurement of aspirin responsiveness or changing the aspirin dose based on platelet function measurements is not recommended at this time [16,59]. Monitoring of aspirin responsiveness is really being conducted only for research purposes at present.

Clopidogrel

Clopidogrel Metabolism

Clopidogrel, a second generation thienopyridine, is a prodrug that requires hepatic conversion to an active metabolite to exert its antiplatelet response. Most of the absorbed clopidogrel (~85–90 %) is hydrolyzed by hepatic carboxylase to an inactive carboxylic acid metabolite, SR26334, whereas the remaining ~10–15 % is rapidly metabolized by hepatic cytochrome (CYP) P450 isoenzymes in a two-step process. In the first step, the thiophene ring of clopidogrel is oxidized to

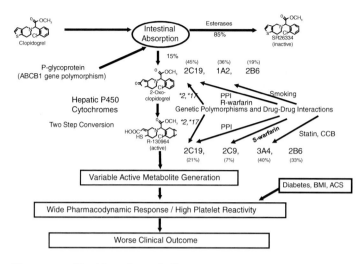

FIGURE 2.5 Clopidogrel metabolism

2-oxo-clopidogrel, which is then converted to a highly unstable active metabolite, R-130964 [60, 61] (Fig. 2.5). R-130964 covalently binds to platelet P2Y$_{12}$ receptor specifically and irreversibly during the passage of platelets through the hepatic circulation resulting in the inhibition of ADP-induced platelet activation and aggregation for the life span of the platelet [62]. Covalent binding of the active metabolite to the P2Y$_{12}$ receptor explains the slow recovery of platelet function following drug withdrawal [63, 64].

Mechanisms Responsible for Clopidogrel Nonreponsiveness

Multiple lines of evidence strongly suggest that variable and insufficient active metabolite generation are the primary explanations for clopidogrel response variability and nonresponsiveness, respectively [65]. Variable levels of active metabolite generation following clopidogrel administration could be explained by: (i) variable or limited intestinal absorption which may be affected by an *ABCB1* gene polymorphism; (ii) functional variability in P450 isoenzyme activity influenced by drug-drug interactions as well as other factors; and (iii) single nucleotide polymorphisms (SNP's) of specific genes encoding CYP450 isoenzymes [66, 67]. Stimulation of CYP3A4 activity by rifampicin and St. Johns Wort, and of CYP1A2 activity by tobacco smoking, have been shown to enhance platelet inhibition induced by clopidogrel [68–70]. The effect of smoking on the antiplatelet effect of clopidogrel has been associated with clinical outcomes, and may in part explain the "smoker's paradox" [71, 72]. Conversely, agents that compete with clopidogrel for CYP and/or inhibit CYP, attenuate the antiplatelet effect of clopidogrel. A diminished pharmacodynamic response to clopidogrel has been observed with co-administration of proton pump inhibitors such as omeprazole, lipophilic statins, and calcium channel blockers that are metabolized by the CYP2C19 and CYP3A4 isoenzymes [73–79]. Although a diminished level of platelet inhibition induced by clopidogrel has been demonstrated in some *ex vivo* studies following co-administration of these agents, the consequence of these interactions with respect to the risk for ischemic event occurrence remains controversial.

Multiple independent studies have demonstrated a link between the presence of genetic polymorphisms associated with suboptimal clopidogrel active metabolite generation (pharmacokinetic measurements), decreased clopidogrel responsiveness as measured by platelet function assays (pharmacodynamic measurements) and adverse clinical outcomes. No single study has conclusively associated all of these parameters in the same patient population.

Recent studies have evaluated the influence of SNPs of the gene encoding CY2C19 as well as SNPs of the p-glycoprotein transporter (ABCB1) gene on clopidogrel response variability and clinical outcomes [67, 80]. In addition to the above mechanisms explaining clopidogrel pharmacodynamic variability, increased body mass index, diabetes mellitus and acute coronary syndromes have also been associated with a diminished antiplatelet response to clopidogrel [80–83]. Finally, noncompliance is an obvious factor which must be excluded in the diagnosis of clopidogrel nonresponsiveness. When attempting to define causality for high platelet reactivity related to the occurrence of clinical events in patients receiving clopidogrel, all of the aforementioned mechanisms should be considered.

The Rationale for Genetic Testing During Clopidogrel Therapy

CYP isoenzyme activity is influenced by single nucleotide polymorphisms (SNPs) resulting in variable and, in some cases, insufficient clopidogrel active metabolite generation leading to resistance and high on treatment platelet reactivity (HPR). There are at least 25 single nucleotide polymorphisms (SNPs) of the gene encoding the CYP2C19 isoenzyme that influence the catalytic activity of the CYP2C19 isoenzyme in a co-dominant (i.e., dose-dependent) manner [84]. The most widely analyzed and most frequent SNPs are CYP2C19*2, a G→A mutation in exon 5 producing an aberrant splice site leading to the complete absence of CYP2C19 activity, and *17 (−806 C→T), a regulatory region variant that has been associated with increased expression and enzymatic activity. The *2 is the most common *loss-of-function (LoF) allele*, with an allelic frequency of approximately ~15 % in Caucasians and African-Americans, and 29–35 % in Asians. *CYP2C19*3* is the second most common *LoF allele*, with an allelic frequency of approximately 2–9 % in Asians but rarely found in other ethnicities. Less common *LoF alleles* include *4, *5, *6, *7, and *8, among others [85]. The *2 loss-of-function and *17 gain-of- function alleles are in linkage disequilibrium (D'=1, $r^2=0.04$) [86, 87].

Less plasma clopidogrel active metabolite exposure (34 % relative reduction, $p<0.001$) and less platelet inhibition (9 % absolute reduction from baseline, $p<0.001$) were demonstrated in healthy carriers of at least one *CY2C19 LOF* allele compared to noncarriers [88]. Poor metabolizers (*2/*2) are

not well represented in most studies due low genotypic frequency. It was reported that, although both *2 and *17 allele
carriage influence ADP-induced platelet aggregation, the
influence of * 2 is more pronounced in patients undergoing
stenting during maintenance therapy. Moreover, for most
patients (those who are not homozygous for either *2 or *17),
HPR cannot be excluded by the results of genotyping in
patients on aspirin and clopidogrel maintenance therapy.
Platelet function is highly variable within diplotype groups
except *2 homozygotes. These data suggest that for most
patients (those who are not homozygous for CYP2C19*2),
genotype fails to identify a large proportion of patients on
maintenance DAPT with HPR. Because both HPR and
CYP2C19 genotype are imperfect correlates of each other
and are predictors of poorer cardiovascular outcomes, genotyping and platelet function testing, together, may provide
complementary information to stratify cardiovascular event
risk in patients on DAPT than either alone [86].

Single Nucleotide Polymorphisms and Clinical Outcomes

In the first genome wide association study, conducted in
healthy Amish subjects, CYP2C19*2 was the only SNP associated with clopidogrel response variability. In this homog-
enous population, a single site in linkage disequilibrium
with (i.e., corresponding to) CYP2C19*2 was found to be
significantly associated with diminished platelet response
($p = 1.5 \times 10^{-13}$), and accounted for only 12 % of the variation
in platelet aggregation to ADP after clopidogrel treatment.
However, clopidogrel response was highly heritable, and
therefore it is possible that non-single nucleotide polymorphisms (e.g., copy number variants, insertions/deletions),
rare variants, or a SNP not included in the analyses may also
contribute to platelet response variability. In a replication
study of PCI patients, carriers of the CYP2C19*2 allele had
a ~2.4x higher cardiovascular event rate compared with

noncarriers [87]. In clopidogrel-treated patients enrolled in the TRITON TIMI-38 study, *LoF* carriers had 1.53x increased risk of primary efficacy outcome of the risk of death from cardiovascular causes, myocardial infarction, or stroke, and 3x increased risk of stent thrombosis as compared with non-carriers [89]. In a collaborative meta-analysis of various clinical trials involving primarily patients who underwent PCI (91 %), an increased risk of the composite end point of CV death, MI or stroke among carriers of 1 *LoF* allele (1.6x) and also carriers of 2 *LoF* alleles (1.8x), as compared with noncarriers was reported. A significantly increased risk of stent thrombosis in both carriers of 1 *LoF* allele (2.7x) and 2 *LoF* alleles (4x) as compared with noncarriers was also observed [90]. It was also reported that patients carrying two *LoF* alleles had a 1.98x higher rate of cardiovascular events than non-carriers among acute myocardial patients and the risk was even higher (3.6x) among patients who underwent PCI [91].

Subsequent retrospective analyses of trials involving mainly non-PCI patients failed to demonstrate a significant association between *CYP2C19 LoF* allele carriage and adverse clinical outcomes. The relation of the gain of function allele (*CYP2C19*17*) carrier status and *ABCB1* genotype to antiplatelet response of clopidogrel and clinical outcomes in clopidogrel-treated patients are inconclusive at this time [92–94]. Most recently, a SNP of the gene encoding paraoxonase-1 (PON-1) has been linked to the pharmacokinetic and pharmacodynamic effects of clopidogrel and stent thrombosis [95]. However, no influence of the *PON-1* polymorphism on platelet reactivity during clopidogrel therapy was reported in subsequent studies [96–98].

Taken together, *LoF* allele carrier status is an important independent predictor of the PD response to clopidogrel and the outcomes of high risk clopidogrel-treated patients who have undergone PCI. The strong relation of carriage to the occurrence of stent thrombosis is noteworthy and is a major rationale for determining the genotype of the PCI patient being considered for, or already treated with, clopidogrel.

Comparison Between Genotyping and Platelet Function Testing

It should be noted that the CYP2C19 isoenzyme is not the only factor determining the antiplatelet response to clopidogrel since, even in genetically-predicted poor metabolizers, some degree of platelet inhibition has been observed where no enzyme activity is expected. It is conceivable that in CYP2C19 poor metabolizers, other isoenzymes, particularly CYP3A4, a very abundant hepatic enzyme, may play an important role in clopidogrel bioactivation. Moreover, clopidogrel metabolism is influenced by concomitantly administered agents such as proton pump inhibitors, calcium channel blockers, warfarin, and cigarette smoke that either inhibit or enhance CYP activity or compete with clopidogrel during hepatic cytochrome P450-mediated metabolism. In addition, demographic variables such as age, renal failure, diabetes, and body mass index also influence the platelet response to ADP by either directly affecting platelet function or by affecting clopidogrel metabolism. The final platelet reactivity phenotype and clinical outcomes of patients treated with clopidogrel are the result of all of these influences. However, genotyping may be more relevant in clopidogrel naive patients to be treated with PCI to determine the optimal initial antiplatelet treatment strategy. Whether genetic testing is complementary to platelet function testing is unknown. A comparison of genetic and platelet function testing is given in Table 2.3.

Rationale for Platelet Function Monitoring During Clopidogrel Therapy: Clopidogrel Response Variability

Clopidogrel response variability was demonstrated by ADP-induced platelet aggregation, and p-selectin and activated GPIIb/IIIa expression assessed at baseline and serially for 30 days following stenting in patients treated with a 300 mg clopidogrel load followed by 75 mg daily therapy. Some patients

TABLE 2.3 Comparison between genotyping and platelet function testing

Genotyping	Platelet function testing
Stable risk factor	Labile risk factor
No method variability	Method variability
Assists in choosing initial prescription	No assistance in choosing initial prescription
Provides "Yes" or "No" readout	Provides continuous readout
Supported by multicenter trial data	Supported by multiregistry data
No proven prospective evidence	No proven prospective evidence
Addressed in guidelines	Addressed in guidelines

had no demonstrable antiplatelet effect i.e., the absolute difference between pre- and post-treatment platelet aggregation was ≤10 % and were regarded as "resistant" (Fig. 2.7) [99]. The prevalence of resistant patients was ~30 % at days 1 and 5 post-stenting, and it fell to 15 % at day 30. In addition, the level of platelet reactivity early after a standard clopidogrel regimen for coronary stenting was critically dependent on the pretreatment reactivity. A similar observation in patients treated with both clopidogrel and prasugrel has been demonstrated by others, suggesting that patients who are hyperresponsive to ADP before treatment are likely to be hyper-responsive to ADP during thienopyridine treatment [100, 101].

There was also a numerical reduction in platelet reactivity observed over time [99]. A similar decrease in the prevalence of high on-treatment platelet reactivity (up to 50 % decrease) at day 30 compared to day 1 post-stenting has been reported in later studies [102, 103]. The reason for this time dependent decrease is still not clear. The time course of platelet reactivity in patients with acute coronary syndromes treated medically is unknown. In a study involving stable coronary artery disease patients, the rates of HPR were similar at 24 h after a

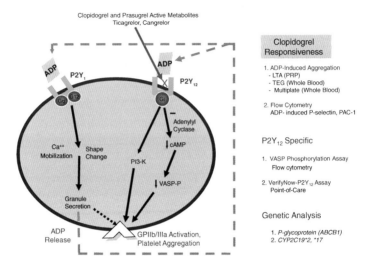

FIGURE 2.6 Laboratory evaluation of clopidogrel responsiveness

600 mg clopidogrel loading dose and after 6 weeks of 75 mg clopidogrel maintenance therapy. In the latter study, platelet reactivity was measured before and after the final maintenance dose; an increase in platelet inhibition (~20 PRU decrease between pre- and post-dosing) was observed at 8 h after the last maintenance dose. These findings indicated an important "booster" effect of the last maintenance induced by new active metabolite generation [64]. Therefore, an estimate of the antiplatelet effect of clopidogrel is influenced by the time of measurement after clopidogrel administration even during the maintenance phase.

Numerous studies utilizing various laboratory methods to assess ADP-induced platelet function (such as turbidimetric aggregation, flow cytometry to measure p-selectin and activated GPIIb/IIIa expression, and vasodilator stimulated phosphoprotein phosphorylation levels) and point-of-care methods (VerifyNow P2Y12 Assay, Platelet Mapping with Thrombelastography and Multiplate analyzer) have been used to demonstrate clopidogrel response variability and resistance (Fig. 2.6) [104–109]. Clopidogrel response variability and resistance are now accepted pharmacodynamic phenomena.

Link Between High Platelet Reactivity and Post-PCI Ischemic/Thrombotic Events

Numerous studies have reported pharmacological "resistance" to clopidogrel as a potential etiology for thrombotic events after PCI (Table 2.4) [37, 104–129]. Barragan et al. first reported an association between post-treatment $P2Y_{12}$ reactivity and the occurrence of thrombotic events (clinical treatment failure) in a case–control study of PCI patients [118]. In the study by Barragan, a platelet reactivity index (PRI) >50 % measured by vasodilator stimulated phosphoprotein (VASP)-phosphorylation assay was associated with stent thrombosis. At the same time Matetzky et al., using aggregometry, observed that patients undergoing primary PCI for STEMI who were in the lowest quartile of clopidogrel responsiveness had the highest rates of ischemic events during follow-up [110].

Subsequently, it was suggested that the level of on-treatment platelet reactivity may be a superior risk predictor compared to the difference between baseline and post-treatment platelet reactivity, since platelet reactivity to ADP was variable before clopidogrel treatment in patients on aspirin therapy [101, 130]. The important relationship between high on-treatment platelet reactivity to ADP as measured by turbidimetric aggregometry and the occurrence of ischemic events in patients treated with stents was first prospectively demonstrated in the Platelet REactivity in Patients And Recurrent Events POST-STENTING (PREPARE POST-STENTING) study (upper quartile, odds ratio 2.6) [106]. In the latter study a threshold of ~50 % maximal periprocedural aggregation (20 μM ADP) was strongly associated with 6-month ischemic event occurrence; the occurrence of ischemic events rarely occurred in patients with aggregation <50 %. These data implied that 50 % maximum aggregation was a therapeutic target for protection from post-PCI thrombotic/ischemic events. In the clopidogrel effect on platelet reactivity in patients with stent thrombosis (CREST) study, ~40 % aggregation (20 μM ADP) was associated with the onset of risk for stent thrombosis occurrence [121]. In a third

TABLE 2.4 Studies linking high on-treatment platelet reactivity to ADP and clopidogrel nonresponsiveness to Post-PCI Adverse Clinical Event Occurrence

Study	Patients (n)	Treatment	Methods	Definition	Clinical relevance
Barragan et al. [108]	PCI (46)	250 mg qd TLP or CLP 75 mg qd	VASP-PRI	>50 % VASP-PRI	↑ stent thrombosis
Gurbel et al. [105, 111, 120]	Elective PCI (192)	300 mg LD + 75 mg qd CLP +/− EPT	5 µM ADP-LTA	HPR = 75 percentile post-PCI aggregation	↑ 6 months post-PCI events, OR = 2.7
Matzesky et al. [155]	PCI-STEMI (60)	300 mg LD + 75 mg qd CLP +/− EPT	5 µM ADP-LTA	Reduction in platelet aggregation upper quartile	↑ 6 months cardiac events
Gurbel et al. [2]	Elective PCI (120)	300 mg LD CLP +/− EPT	5 µM ADP-LTA	Mean periprocedural platelet aggregation > 50 %	↑ periprocedural myonecrosis
Gurbel et al. [106, 111, 121]	Elective PCI (200)	300/600 mg LD CLP +/− EPT	5 µM ADP-LTA	Mean periprocedural platelet aggregation > 40 %	↑ periprocedural myonecrosis
Bliden et al. [105]	Elective PCI (100)	75 mg qd CLP	5 µM ADP-LTA	>50 % platelet aggregation	↑ 1 year post-PCI events

Lev et al. [36]	Elective PCI (150)	300 mg CLP LD	5 and 20 μMADP-LTA	Baseline – post-treatment aggregation ≤10 %	↑ periprocedural myonecrosis
Blindt et al. [113]	High risk for ST –PCI (99)	75 mg qd for 6 months	VASP-PRI (72–96 after stenting)	>48 % PRI (ROC)	↑ 6 month ST
Cuisset et al. [114]	NSTE-ACS-PCI (190)	600 mg CLP LD >6 h before PCI	10 μM ADP-LTA VASP-PRI	HPR: >70 % Post-treatment LTA	↑ periprocedural myonecrosis
Frere et al. [115]	NSTE-ACS-PCI (195)	600 mg CLP LD >6 h before PCI	10 μM ADP-LTA	HPR (ROC): >70 % post-treatment LTA >53 % VASP-PRI	↑ 30 d post-PCI events MACE+stroke
Geisler et al. [116]	CAD-PCI (379)	600 mg CLP LD >6 h before PCI	20 μM ADP-LTA	Clopidogrel low responders = <30 % platelet inhibition	↑ 3 months MACE and death OR=4.9
Geisler et al. [117]	CAD-PCI (1092)	600 mg CLP LD>6 h before PCI +75 mg qd	20 μM ADP-LTA Residual aggregation measured after 5 min	Upper quartile	↑ 30 days MACE

(continued)

TABLE 2.4 (continued)

Study	Patients (n)	Treatment	Methods	Definition	Clinical relevance
Hochholzer et al. [118]	Elective PCI (802)	600 mg CLP LD >2 h before PCI +75 mg qd	5 μM ADP-LTA Residual aggregation measured after 5 min	Platelet aggregation above median	↑ 30 days MACE, OR = 6.7
Price et al. [119]	PCI (380)	600 mg CLP LD >12 h before PCI or 75 mg qd > 5 days	VerifyNow P2Y12 assay	HPR = post-treatment ≥235 PRU (ROC)	↑ 6 months post-PCI events including ST
Gurbel et al. [120]	Elective PCI (297)	300 or 600 mg LD/75 mg qd CLP +/– EPT	5 and 20 μM ADP-LTA	HPR = post-procedural (ROC) >46 % 5 μM ADP >59 % 20 μM ADP	↑ 2-year ischemic events 5 μM ADP OR = 3.9 20 μM ADP OR = 3.8
Gurbel et al. [106, 111, 121]	Stenting (120)	75 mg qd CLP >5 days	5 and 20 μM ADP-LTA	HPR >75 percentile of platelet reactivity 5 μM ADP = 50 % 20 μM ADP = 65 %	↑ stent thrombosis
Buonamici et al. [122]	PCI-DES (804)	600 mg LD 75 mg qd for 6 months	10 μM ADP-LTA	HPR ≥70 % aggregation	↑ stent thrombosis HR = 3.08
Bonello et al. [123]	PCI-stenting (144)	300 mg LD >24 h	VASP-PRI	>50 % PRI (ROC)	↑ 6 months Post-PCI MACE

Cuisset et al. [124]	PCI-SA (120)	600 mg LD ≥12 h before PCI	VerifyNow P2Y12 assay	↑ platelet reactivity	↑ post-PCI myonecrosis
Migliorini et al. [125]	PCI-DES-ULMD (215)	600 mg LD + 75 mg qd for 12 months	10 µM ADP-LTA	HPR- ≥70 % aggregation	↑ 3 years cardiac death and ST HR CV death = 3.82 HR ST = 3.69
Marcucci et al. [126]	PCI-ACS (683)	600 mg LD + 75 mg qd	VerifyNow P2Y12 assay	HPR ≥240 PRU	12-month ischemic event HR CV death = 2.55 HR nonfatal MI = 3.36
Patti et al. [127]	PCI (160)	600 mg LD or 75 mg qd > 5 days	VerifyNow P2Y12 assay	HPR ≥240 PRU (Pre-PCI)	↑ 1 month major cardiovascular event occurrence
Cuisset et al. [128, 147]	NSTEMI-Stenting (598)	600 mg LD ≥12 h before PCI	10 µM ADP-LTA VASP-PRI	>67 % Aggregation (ROC)	↑ Stent thrombosis

(continued)

Table 2.4 (continued)

Study	Patients (n)	Treatment	Methods	Definition	Clinical relevance
Breet et al. [129]	Elective PCI (1,069)	75 mg qd >5 days	5 and 20 μM ADP-LTA	>42.9 % 5 μM ADP (ROC)	OR for 1 year death, MI, ST and stroke 5 μM ADP =2.09 20 μM ADP =2.05
		300 mg LD >1d	VerifyNow P2Y12 20 μM	>64.5 % 20uM ADP	VerifyNow =2.53
		600 mg LD >4 h	ADP-plateleworks Before PCI	>236 PRU 80.5 % plateleworks	Plateleworks =2.22
Sibbing et al. [129]	PCI-DES (1608)	600 mg LD before PCI	6.4 μM ADP-multiplate analyzer	Upper quintile (>416 AU*min) (ROC)	↑ 1 month definite stent thrombosis (OR=9.4)
Bonello et al. [65]	PCI-stenting (162)	600 mg repeated dose till PRI <50 %	VASP-PRI	<50 % VASP-PRI	↓ 1 month-ischemic event

Bonello et al. [150]	PCI-stenting (214)	600 mg repeated dose till PRI <50 %	VASP-PRI	<50 % VASP-PRI	↓ Early stent thrombosis and MACE (OR=9.4)
Valgimigli et al. [151]	Elective PCI (1,277)	600 mg LD before PCI	VerifyNow aspirin and P2Y12 assay	>235 PRU >550 ARU	↑ 3- day post-PCI and 1 year outcome

LTA light transmittance aggregometry, *ADP* adenosine diphosphate, *PCI* percutaneous intervention, *MACE* major adverse clinical events, *VASP-PRI* vasodilator stimulated phosphoprotein – platelet reactivity index, *PRU* P2Y12 reaction units, *MI* myocardial infarction, *AU* aggregation units, *DES* drug eluting stent, *NSTEMI* non ST segment elevated myocardial infarction, *ROC* receiver operating characteristic curve, *LD* loading dose, *qd* once daily, *OR* odds ratio, *AA* arachidonic acid, *ST* stent thrombosis, *TL* ticlopidine, *CLP* clopidogrel, *ULMD* unprotected left main disease

study, ~40 % pre-procedural platelet aggregation (5 μM ADP) among patients receiving long-term clopidogrel and aspirin therapy before stenting was associated with 12 month ischemic event occurrence [105]. Price demonstrated that patients with post-treatment reactivity >235 PRU (~upper quartile) had significantly higher rates of cardiovascular death (2.8 % vs. 0 %, p = 0.04) and stent thrombosis (4.6 % vs. 0 %, p = 0.004) [119]. Interestingly, in the largest prospective trial of personalized antiplatelet therapy, GRAVITAS, immunity to ischemic event occurrence was associated with <170 PRU as measured by VerifyNow [102]. Sibbing et al. using the Multiplate analyzer, demonstrated that low responders as indicated by upper quintile (~482 AU*min) had a significantly higher risk of definite stent thrombosis and a higher mortality rate within 30 days compared with normal responders [109]. These studies have primarily used a single measurement of reactivity determined either immediately before PCI or at the time of hospital discharge. A recent consensus statement proposed cutoff values based on receiver operating characteristic curve analysis for different platelet function assays to be used in future studies of personalized antiplatelet therapy (Table 2.5) (65, 109, 119, 120, 123). A recent patient based meta-analysis of studies employing the VerifyNow point-of-care assay lends further support for the potential role of monitoring of $P2Y_{12}$ receptor blocker therapy as a diagnostic marker [132]. The latter data were strongly supported by results from the ADAPT-DES (Assessment of Dual AntiPlatelet Therapy with Drug-Eluting Stents) trial, an investigation (n > 8,000) of the relation of post-PCI platelet reactivity measured by the VerifyNow assay to thrombotic events. In ADAPT-DES, patients with >208 PRU (P2Y12 reaction units) had a three-fold adjusted hazard for the occurrence of 30 day stent thrombosis [133].

Taken together, these data suggest that adequate protection against ischemic events with aspirin and clopidogrel therapy might be achieved by overall low to moderate levels of post-treatment platelet reactivity in the majority of patients. Many subsequent studies have confirmed the

TABLE 2.5 Selected studies linking high on-treatment platelet reactivity to ischemic events based on receiver operating characteristic curve analysis with a specific cut off value

Study	Assay	Cut-off value	Endpoint
Price et al. [119]	VerifyNow P2Y12 assay	>235 PRU	6 months Post-PCI CVD + MI + stent thrombosis
Gurbel et al. [120]	LTA	>46 % 5 μM ADP	2 years post-PCI MACE
		>59 % 20 μM ADP	
Bonello et al. [123]	VASP-PRI	>50 % PRI	6 months Post-PCI MACE
Sibbing et al. [76, 109]	Multiplate analyzer-ADP	>468 AU*min 6.4 μM ADP	30 day stent thrombosis

LTA light transmittance aggregometry, *ADP* adenosine diphosphate, *PCI* percutaneous intervention, *MACE* major adverse clinical events, *VASP-PRI* vasodilator stimulated phosphoprotein – platelet reactivity index, *PRU* P2Y12 reaction units, *MI* myocardial infarction, *AU* aggregation units

direct relationship between the level of platelet reactivity and post–PCI ischemic event occurrence using the following assays: VASP-phosphorylation, conventional aggregation, and VerifyNow and the Multiplate analyzer. These studies have consistently demonstrated that high on -treatment platelet reactivity is an important independent risk factor for the occurrence of thrombotic/ischemic events after PCI [65].

High Platelet Reactivity Defined by ROC Curve Analysis

Studies have emerged that have used receiver operating characteristic (ROC) curve analysis to define a threshold or cut-point of on-treatment platelet reactivity associated with the optimal combination of sensitivity and specificity to identify thrombotic/ischemic risk. It should be noted that such cut-points may depend on the subset of patients studied. In fact, to date, cut off values have been mainly investigated in patients undergoing PCI and different targets may be obtained in other settings depending on patient management or baseline risk profile. The consistent findings across multiple investigations support the crucial role of HPR in the etiology of ischemic events after PCI, including stent thrombosis and suggest the existence of a threshold level of platelet reactivity below which ischemic events may be prevented. The observed cut-off values for platelet reactivity noted above had a very high negative predictive value for thrombotic/ischemic event occurrence, an observation of potential great clinical importance. However, the positive predictive value is fairly low for all assays. This is consistent with the fact that, although a major determinant of thrombotic events, high on-treatment platelet reactivity is not the sole factor responsible for these events [65].

Recently, in the do platelet function assays predict clinical outcomes in clopidogrel pre-treated patients undergoing elective PCI (POPULAR) study, investigators evaluated the utility of multiple platelet function assays in predicting the 1 year outcome of death, myocardial infarction, stent thrombosis and stroke in 1,069 consecutive patients treated with clopidogrel following elective coronary stent implantation. In this large, prospective, observational study, HPR cutpoints of 42.9 % maximal aggregation induced by 5 µM ADP, and 64.5 % by 20 µM ADP LTA; 236 PRU measured by VerifyNow-P2Y12 assay; and 80.5 % aggregation by Plateletworks all correlated with the occurrence of the composite primary endpoint with an area under the curve (AUC) of ~0.62 for each assay. The addition of high on-treatment platelet reactivity as measured by the above noted platelet assays to classical clinical and procedural risk factors improved the AUC to ~0.73 [129]. Similarly, in another study of 1,092 stable angina and patients presenting with an acute coronary syndrome treated with stenting, 30 day ischemic event occurrence was significantly associated with the upper tertile of ADP-induced platelet reactivity measured following the loading dose. In addition, presentation with an acute coronary syndrome, reduced LV-function, diabetes mellitus, renal failure (creatinine >1.5 mg/dL) and age >65 years significantly influenced on-treatment platelet reactivity. Moreover, in a factor-weighed model, HPR risk was increased by these demographic factors [103]. These preliminary results supported an earlier hypothesis that a comprehensive algorithm including clinical as well as laboratory findings (platelet reactivity and genotype) should be considered in future personalized antiplatelet therapy investigations to optimize outcomes.

Platelet Function Monitoring and Avoidance of Bleeding: A Therapeutic Window for P2Y$_{12}$ Inhibitors

Similar to the upper bound platelet reactivity cutoff associated with ischemic event occurrence, there may be lower platelet reactivity cutoff below which the risk for ischemic event occurrence may be minimal whereas bleeding risk may be high [134]. The latter observation may be important during therapy with new P2Y$_{12}$ receptor blockers that are

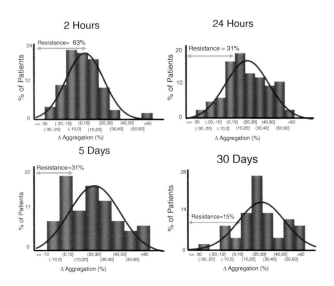

FIGURE 2.7 Demonstration of clopidogrel nonresponsiveness (Adapted from Gurbel et al. [98])

associated with consistently greater platelet inhibition than clopidogrel. (Fig. 2.7) [134]. In the Clopidogrel in Unstable angina to prevent Recurrent Events (CURE) trial, dual antiplatelet therapy was associated with a 38 % increased relative risk of major bleeding compared to aspirin mono-therapy [135]. In the TRITON-TIMI 38 trial, prasugrel treat-ment was associated with a 32 % and 52 % increased relative risk of non- CABG related TIMI major and life-threatening bleeding, respectively [136]. Similarly, in the PLATO trial, there was 27 % increase in non-CABG TIMI major bleeding associated with ticagrelor therapy compared to clopidogrel therapy [137]. The discordance between lower ischemic endpoints and higher bleeding rates during treatment with more potent antiplatelet regimens observed in clinical trials (clopidogrel + aspirin vs. aspirin, prasugrel/ticagrelor + aspi-rin vs. clopidogrel + aspirin) suggest that improved clinical efficacy will be accompanied by reduced safety in clinical practice (Fig. 2.8).

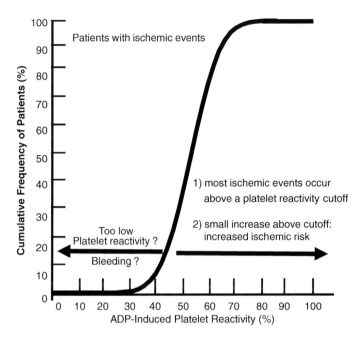

FIGURE 2.8 The concept of a therapeutic window for $P2Y_{12}$ blockade

In this line, three recent preliminary translational research studies support the concept of a lower platelet reactivity cutoff for bleeding risk in patients treated with PCI. An increased responsiveness to clopidogrel measured by ADP-induced platelet aggregation using multiple electrode aggregometry (MEA) was associated with a 3.5 increased risk of procedure related major bleeding in patients (n = 2,533) undergoing PCI [138]. In the latter study, more bleeding events were observed in patients with <188 AU*minutes as measured by Multiplate analyzer whereas the same investigators demonstrated the significant association of ischemic events in patients with >468 AU* min. In another study, ≤86 PRU and ≥239 PRU as measured by the VerifyNow P2Y12 assay were significantly associated with 1 month bleeding events and ischemic event occurrence, respectively in 507 patients undergoing PCI [103].

Based on receiver operating characteristic curve analysis, it was demonstrated that >47 ADP-induced platelet-fibrin clot strength (MA_{ADP}) as measured by thrombelastography with the Platelet Mapping assay was associated with 3 year ischemic event occurrence whereas ≤31 MA_{ADP} was associated with the occurrence of bleeding events in 225 patients undergoing stenting treated with aspirin and clopidogrel [139]. Similarly, other observational studies indicated that very low platelet reactivity was associated with bleeding (Table 2.6) [103, 138–147]. The concept of a "therapeutic window" of P2Y12 receptor reactivity associated with both ischemic event occurrence (upper threshold) and bleeding risk (lower threshold) has been proposed similar to the international normalized ratio (INR) range used for coumadin therapy, potentially allowing for personalization of antiplatelet therapy [134].

Personalized Antiplatelet Therapy-Preliminary Prospective Studies

Following the demonstration of a link between high on-treatment platelet reactivity in patients undergoing PCI and thrombotic/ischemic events, several studies have aimed to lower the level of platelet reactivity by modifying therapy. These studies have demonstrated that platelet reactivity to ADP on standard clopidogrel therapy can be lowered by using higher loading or maintenance doses of clopidogrel, the addition of cilostazol, switching to more potent alternative $P2Y_{12}$ receptor blockers such as prasugrel or ticagrelor, and by adding elinogrel or GPIIb/IIIa inhibitors [148–159]. An improved outcome with altered therapy was observed in some of these studies [148–151].

In two small multicenter trials that employed the VASP-phosphorylation assay, tailored incremental loading doses of clopidogrel further reduced on-treatment platelet reactivity below the above noted threshold and were effective in reducing subsequent major adverse cardiovascular events without increasing Thrombolysis in Myocardial Infarction

TABLE 2.6 Selected studies linking platelet function measurement to bleeding

Study	Patients	Platelet function assay	Bleeding outcome
CABG patients			
Chen et al. [27, 139]	Patients treated with clopidogrel within 6 days of CABG (n=45)	ADP-induced PA	<40 % pre-heparin ADP-induced platelet aggregation predicted 92 % severe coagulopathies requiring multiple transfusions
Mahla et al. [140]	CABG patients treated with and without clopidogrel (n=192)	MA-ADP Platelet mapping Assay	Stratifying clopidogrel treated patients based on preoperative assessment of clopidogrel response results in similar peri-operative bleeding as compared to clopidogrel naïve patients
Reece et al. [141]	CABG patients (n=44)	ADP-and TRAP-induced PA by LTA and MEA	PA measured by MEA was reduced in transfused patients compared to not transfused

Table 2.6 (continued)

Study	Patients	Platelet function assay	Bleeding outcome
Kwak et al. [142]	CABG patients (n=100)	MA-ADP Platelet mapping Assay	70 % platelet inhibition was associated with post-operative transfusion requirement in ROC analysis (AUC=0.77. 95 %; CI=0.67–0.87; p<0.001)
Ranucci et al. [143]	On-pump CABG patients treated with clopidogrel (n=87)	ADP-and TRAP-induced PA MEA	ADP-induced PA 31U is associated with postoperative bleeding in RCO analysis (AUC=0.71.95 %; CI=0.59–0.83; p=0.013)
Post-PCI patients			
Sibbing et al. [137]	PCI patients pre-treated with 600 mg clopidogrel (n=2,533)	ADP-induced PA with MEA	<188 AU min is an independent predictor in-hospital of major bleeding (OR=3.5, 95 % CI=1.6–7.3; p=0.001)

Reference	Population	Assay	Findings
Gurbel et al. [138, 157, 158]	Post-PCI, (n=225), 3 year outcome	Post-PCI TEG-Platelet mapping Assay	All Major Bleeding Events occurred within the 1st Quartile of MA-ADP(929) ROC for bleeding=31 MAADP
	Elective or ACS pts –PCI on CLP and ASA (n=346)	VASP assay	Lower VASP index=In-hospital major bleeding (33 +/−22 % vs. 51 +/−22)
Campo et al. [101]	Post-PCI, (n=300) 1 year follow-up	Pre-PCI VerifyNow P2Y12 assay	>238 PRU Ischemic events <86 bleeding events
Patti et al. [145]	Post-PCI (n=310)	Pre-PCI VerifyNow P2Y12 assay	<189 PRU=30 day major bleeding
Cuisset et al. [126, 146]	NSTE-ACS (n=597)–1 month follow-up	ADP-induced PA VASP	<40 % post-treatment PA (hyper-responders, first quartile) had higher risk of 30 day TIMI major and minor bleeding

PCI percutaneous coronary interventions, *ADP* adenosine diphosphate, *PA* platelet aggregation, *MEA* multiple electrode analyser, *AU* arbitrary units, *CI* confidence interval, *NSTE-ACS* non-ST segment elevationacute coronary syndrome, *TIMI* thrombolysis in myocardial infarction, *CABG* coronary artery bypass grafting surgery, *ROC* receiver operating characteristic curve, *AUC* area under the curve

(TIMI) major or minor bleedings. However it must be noted that 8–14 % of patients remained with HPR to clopidogrel even after repeated loading doses of 600 mg [148, 149]. Similarly, following these findings, two other studies have suggested that the selective administration of platelet glycoprotein (GP) IIb/IIIa receptor blockers to patients undergoing elective PCI who were identified as having high on-treatment platelet reactivity following an oral clopidogrel loading dose was effective in reducing both 30 day and 1 year post-PCI ischemic events without increased bleeding rates [150, 151]. These studies were the first to suggest that the cut off value identifying patients at increased risk of thrombotic events could be used to tailor therapy effectively and, in turn, lead to improved outcomes.

The GRAVITAS trial was the first large scale investigation of personalized antiplatelet therapy in the elective PCI patient [102]. Patients with HPR were treated with either a 600 mg extra loading dose given the day after stenting followed by twice the standard-dose of clopidogrel maintenance therapy or standard-dose clopidogrel therapy for 6 months. In addition, a group of patients without HPR were treated with standard-dose clopidogrel therapy. High dose clopidogrel treatment was ineffective in reducing the 6-month composite of ischemic event occurrence (cardiovascular death, non-fatal myocardial infarction, and stent thrombosis); both HPR groups had an unexpectedly low event rate (2.3 %). Several reasons were proposed for the neutral results of GRAVITAS. The most unlikely is that HPR identified following PCI is a risk indicator and not a modifiable risk factor. A credible argument against the latter were the results from large scale clinical trials of ACS patients demonstrating that treatment with $P2Y_{12}$ inhibitors associated with more potent platelet inhibition than clopidogrel produced lower ischemic event rates than clopidogrel treatment. Another is that high dose clopidogrel was a suboptimal remedy to overcome HPR. In GRAVITAS, high-dose clopidogrel reduced the prevalence of HPR at 30 days in only 60 % of patients. In a study with an event rate as low as GRAVITAS, only treatment with a highly effective remedy to reduce HPR would have provided the greatest likelihood to produce a positive clinical trial result. Finally, the cutoff for HPR may have been too high [160]. Subsequent analyses from GRAVITAS have demonstrated the clustering of events above and below the HPR cutoff of 230 P2Y12 reactivity units (PRUs) and that "responders" had events that clustered just below 230 PRU. In a time-covariate Cox regression analysis of on-treatment platelet reactivity, PRU <208 was an independent predictor of event free survival at 60 days (HR=0.23, 95 % CI=0.05–0.98, p=0.047) and strongly trended to be an independent predictor at 6 months (HR=0.54, 95 % CI=0.28–1.04, p=0.06) [161]. These findings are particularly important given the very low event rate observed in GRAVITAS [102]. In the recently presented Testing platelet Reactivity In patients underGoing elective stent placement on clopidogrel to Guide alternative thErapy with pRasugrel (TRIGER-PCI) study, a 10 mg daily dose of prasugrel was effective in reducing on-treatment platelet reactivity compared to 75 mg daily dose clopidogrel [162]. The latter personalized antiplatelet trial used >208 PRU a cutpoint for HPR. However, the study was terminated early for futility because of extremely low event rates.

At this time many important issues remain unresolved. The HPR threshold mentioned in the consensus statement was determined by ROC analysis and is only applicable to the PCI population. However, based on the group of patients from GRAVITAS treated with standard dose clopidogrel, an even lower threshold defining HPR (~170 PRU) was associated with optimal identification of patients destined to experience ischemic event occurrence. It was suggested that this "immunity to thrombosis" cutoff should be considered as the new therapeutic target in the PCI patient [163]. During the early phase of ACS and/or PCI, platelet activity is greatest, and the prevalence of clopidogrel nonresponsiveness level is higher. At that time a potent antiplatelet regimen may provide the greatest net clinical benefit (reduction in ischemic events that outweighs the risk of bleeding events) whereas at time points further downstream from the ACS event, less intense antiplatelet effects may be desirable. The optimal HPR threshold at ~30 days may therefore differ from the acute threshold during the index ACS hospitalization. The HPR cutoffs proposed thus far are based on a single measurement [either before PCI (mostly European studies) or before discharge (American studies)]. Longitudinal platelet function measurements have never been done in a large scale antiplatelet therapy trial in ACS patients. Knowledge gained from such an analysis will enhance our understanding of the relationship between platelet reactivity, and ischemic and bleeding event occurrences.

It should be taken into consideration that the currently accepted HPR cutoff values have been associated in many studies with modestly increased odds ratios for ischemic event occurrence and are associated with high negative predictive values and low positive predictive values (PPV). However, given the overall low prevalence of thrombotic events in these studies, the low PPV is understandable. Moreover, there is debate about whether diagnostic test statistics were appropriately used to describe the utility of prognostic tests, such as platelet function tests. The current data indicate that although platelet reactivity plays a major role in ischemic event occurrence (up to 50 % of the attributable risk of 30 day stent thrombosis in ADEPT-DES), other factors including demographic and clinical factors must be taken into consideration to optimally define the patients at greatest risk. Along this line, recent studies also suggest that adding clinical variables and genotype to platelet reactivity measurements (combined risk factor) will improve risk prediction [129, 164].

Thus far, the relation of platelet reactivity to bleeding has not been investigated in a systematic fashion within a large scale prospective clinical trial. The ability to evaluate bleeding susceptibility is highly relevant, as it may enable the tailoring of antiplatelet therapy to enhance the risk-benefit balance and net clinical benefit during DAPT particularly with potent P2Y12 receptor blocker therapy.

Role of Platelet Function Measurement in Patients Undergoing Coronary Artery Bypass Surgery (CABG)

Thienopyridines (clopidogrel and prasugrel) and aspirin are irreversible inhibitors that are associated with an increased risk of bleeding especially among high-risk patients. Bleeding is a major clinical concern in patients on dual antiplatelet therapy requiring immediate CABG. Current guidelines recommend withholding clopidogrel for at least 5 days and prasugrel at least 7 days before CABG in order to limit blood loss and transfusions (class I recommendation, level of evidence C) [165–167]. In addition, the FDA recommended 5 days of withdrawal from ticagrelor therapy before CABG [168]. Since approximately 8–30 % of patients treated with clopidogrel exhibit a limited or no antiplatelet response, these patients may be eligible for CABG based on platelet function measurements at a time earlier than 5 days after cessation of therapy. Moreover, variability exists in the recovery of platelet function following withdrawal of clopidogrel treatment. Serial preoperative measurements of platelet function may allow patients to undergo CABG earlier than 5 days without an increased risk of bleeding and thus decrease hospitalization time.

It was demonstrated that during routine coronary artery surgery, patients who were transfused exhibited significantly less platelet aggregation as measured by the Multiplate analyzer compared to patients who were not transfused (ADP induced aggregation 18 U vs. 29 U, $p = 0.01$) [142]. Similarly an association between clopidogrel responsiveness measured by the Multiplate analyzer and bleeding was demonstrated in patients undergoing off-pump and also on-pump cardiac surgery with recent clopidogrel exposure [143, 169]. Thrombelastography (TEG) based transfusion algorithms have been demonstrated to reduce transfusion requirements in patients undergoing CABG [170, 171]. Moreover, the addition of TEG measurements (maximum thrombin-induced platelet-fibrin clot strength) to an existing risk prediction model significantly improved the risk stratification for excessive blood loss in patients undergoing on-pump cardiac surgery [172]. Chen et al. were the first to demonstrate an association between platelet aggregation measured by LTA and CABG related bleeding in patients on clopidogrel undergoing first time on-pump CABG. Unadjusted for potential pre- and intra-operative confounders, a pre-heparin ADP induced aggregation less than 40 % corresponding to 60 % platelet inhibition predicted 92 % of cases needing multiple transfusions [140]. The prospective Time BAsed StRateGy to REduce Clopidogrel AssociaTed Bleeding During CABG (TARGET CABG) study, demonstrated that stratifying clopidogrel treated patients based on preoperative assessment of clopidogrel response and timing surgery according to clopidogrel response resulted in similar peri-operative bleeding as compared to clopidogrel naïve patients undergoing elective first time on-pump CABG [141]. In this study pre-operative clopidogrel response was measured by TEG with Platelet Mapping. Surgery was scheduled with no delay in those with a maximum amplitude (MA_{ADP}) >50 mm, within 3–5 days in those with an MA_{ADP} 35–50 mm, and after 5 days in those with an MA_{ADP} <35 mm. These data suggested that delays in surgery may be obviated by preoperatively measuring platelet function and that timing surgery appropriately thereby reduces hospital costs [141]. The results from TARGET CABG require confirmation in a larger investigation.

Monitoring of Antiplatelet Therapy in the Medically Managed ACS Patient

There have been no randomized prospective trials focused exclusively on the use of DAPT in medically managed ACS patients. Antiplatelet therapy monitoring to study the relation of HPR and genotype to clinical outcome in these patients is completely unknown. Moreover, the stability of the HPR phenotype in medically managed ACS patients is very poorly understood as there is no information in patients managed without PCI. Finally, the relation of platelet reactivity and genotype to bleeding risk has been much less studied as compared to the relation to ischemic event occurrence.

The targeted platelet inhibition to clarify the optimal strategy to medically manage acute coronary syndromes (TRILOGY-ACS) study is a global phase III, double-blind, double-dummy, parallel-group randomized-controlled trial comparing prasugrel, a novel thienopyridine platelet inhibitor, with clopidogrel among patients who are medically-managed for a non-ST elevation (NSTE) ACS. The study will enroll approximately 10,300 subjects at 800 sites globally (7,800 subjects <75 years of age and a maximum enrollment of 2,500 subjects ≥75 years of age). Approximately one third of the TRILOGY-ACS study population will be enrolled in the platelet function substudy (n=3,433); these patients will have platelet function assessed with the Accumetrics VerifyNow® P2Y12 and Aspirin assays at multiple time-points throughout the study. In contrast to the preponderance of studies investigating platelet reactivity among patients undergoing PCI, TRILOGY-ACS will provide the unique opportunity to study serial platelet reactivity among patients with ACS who are managed without in-hospital revascularization and examine the relation of reactivity preceding ischemic event occurrence. The TRILOGY-ACS platelet function substudy will be the largest conducted within a major large scale clinical trial and will approximately triple the enrollment of most of the largest platelet function studies conducted thus far [173].

Guidelines

Persistent ischemic event occurrence and the irrefutable demonstration of clopidogrel antiplatelet response variability are two potent arguments against the widely practiced "non-selective" or "one-size-fits- all" strategy of clopidogrel therapy. Observational studies conducted in thousands of patients have led to an international consensus that high-on treatment platelet reactivity to ADP (HPR) is a major risk factor for post-percutaneous coronary intervention (PCI) ischemic event occurrence [65]. Moreover, recent American and European guidelines have given a Class IIb recommendation to perform either platelet function testing (level of evidence B) or genotyping (level of evidence C) if the results of testing may alter management [165, 166, 174]. Furthermore, the Society of Thoracic Surgeons gave a Class IIb recommendation for platelet function testing to determine the timing of surgery in patients on clopidogrel therapy (level of evidence C) [167]. These recommendations for personalizing antiplatelet therapy are unprecedented and are an acknowledgement that a significant body of data supporting testing have accrued in the literature.

Future

Non-selective administration of antiplatelet therapy contradicts common practice in cardiovascular medicine where a measurable drug effect is mandated and, if the response is suboptimal, an alternative strategy is warranted. It is indisputable that HPR and *LoF* carrier status are associated with a significant increase in ischemic risk in PCI patients treated with clopidogrel and this is not surprising given the central role of the ADP-P2Y12 interaction in the genesis of coronary thrombosis. The primary goal of platelet function testing is to identify the patient who is suboptimally responsive and adjust therapy accordingly in order to prevent the catastrophic events of myocardial infarction and stent thrombosis. Genotyping predicts who is at risk of being suboptimally responsive, but does not replace functional testing. It is unreasonable to expect that tests predictive of complex future events such as the occurrence of ischemic events in patients with cardiovascular disease will perform with the same specificity as tests diagnostic of events that have already occurred or are evolving at the time of testing.

Although we don't yet have conclusive evidence from a definitive large scale randomized trial that personalized antiplatelet therapy improves patient outcomes, the evidence is strong enough now to recommend genotyping and phenotyping in the high risk PCI patient. Moreover, conducting the "definitive" randomized personalized antiplatelet therapy trial now may be delicate. Investigators may be reluctant to randomly assign their patients to a less pharmacodynamically effective therapy. A better understanding of the causes of treatment failure potentially will facilitate targeted and optimal inhibition of novel platelet receptors and coagulation factors. Antiplatelet therapy, as a primary therapeutic strategy inhibiting critical pathophysiologic mechanisms, will lead the way in the field of personalization. On the horizon are point-of-care devices that will provide rapid information about genotype and these devices are now available to determine platelet function. There are many gaps in our knowledge regarding the role of platelet function and genetic testing to optimize anti-platelet therapy including (1) no information on stable coronary disease patients, (2) no information on the relation of phenotype to events in medically managed ACS patients, (3) few data on the relation of long term platelet reactivity to both ischemic and bleeding events, (4) preliminary data only on the relation of phenotype and genotype to bleeding, (5) limited data on the utility of combining genotype and phenotype data for prognosis, (6) uncertainty regarding the variability of platelet function over time, (7) limited data relating platelet function to clinical outcomes in a major clinical trial of antiplatelet therapy, and most importantly, (8) limited evidence from a large scale trial that personalization of antiplatelet therapy enhances efficacy and improves safety. Much greater focus on the relation between on-treatment platelet reactivity and bleeding will need to be given in order to establish whether a therapeutic window for $P2Y_{12}$ blockers exists [134]. Although we don't yet have conclusive evidence from a large scale randomized trial(s) that personalized antiplatelet therapy improves patient outcomes, a Class IIb recommendation has been given in the European and American guidelines to perform genotyping or phenotyping in high risk PCI patients if a change in antiplatelet therapy will ensue based on the test results [165, 166, 174].

References

1. Gurbel PA, Tantry US. Combination antithrombotic therapies. Circulation. 2010;121:569–83.
2. Gurbel PA, Bliden KP, Hayes KM, Tantry U. Platelet activation in myocardial ischemic syndromes. Expert Rev Cardiovasc Ther. 2004;2:535–45.
3. Becker RC, Meade TW, Berger PB, et al. American college of chest physicians. The primary and secondary prevention of coronary artery disease: American college of chest physicians evidence-based clinical practice guidelines (8th edition). Chest. 2008;133:776S–814.
4. Tantry US, Bliden KP, Gurbel PA. Resistance to antiplatelet drugs: current status and future research. Expert Opin Pharmacother. 2005;6:2027–45.
5. Gurbel PA, Tantry US. Do platelet function testing and genotyping improve outcome in patients treated with antithrombotic agents?: platelet function testing and genotyping improve outcome in patients treated with antithrombotic agents. Circulation. 2012;125(10):1276–87; discussion 1287.
6. Antithrombotic Trialists' collaboration: collaborative meta-analysis of randomised trials of antiplatelet therapy for prevention of death, myocardial infarction, and stroke in high risk patients. BMJ 2002;324:71–86.
7. Mehta SR, Tanguay JF, Eikelboom JW, et al. CURRENT-OASIS 7 trial investigators. Double-dose versus standard-dose clopidogrel and high-dose versus low-dose aspirin in individuals undergoing percutaneous coronary intervention for acute coronary syndromes (CURRENT-OASIS 7): a randomised factorial trial. Lancet. 2010;376:1233–43.
8. Tantry US, Mahla E, Gurbel PA. Aspirin resistance. Prog Cardiovasc Dis. 2009;52:141–52.
9. Loll PJ, Picot D, Garavito RM. The structural basis of aspirin activity inferred from the crystal structure of inactivated prostaglandin H_2 synthase. Nat Struct Biol. 1995;2:637–43.
10. Chiang N, Serhan CN. Aspirin triggers formation of anti-inflammatory mediators: new mechanism for an old drug. Discov Med. 2004;4:470–5.
11. Di Nino G, Silver MJ, Murphy S. Monitoring the entry of new platelets into circulation after ingestion of aspirin. Blood. 1983;61:1081.

12. Reilly IA, FitzGerald GA. Inhibition of thromboxane formation in vivo and ex vivo: implications for therapy with platelet inhibitory drugs. Blood. 1987;69:180–6.

13. Patrignani P. Aspirin insensitive eicosanoid biosynthesis in cardiovascular disease. Thromb Res. 2003;110:281–6.

14. Rocca B, Secchiero P, Ciabattoni G, et al. Cyclooxygenase-2 expression is induced during human megakaryopoiesis and characterizes newly formed platelets. Proc Natl Acad Sci USA. 2002;99:7634–9.

15. Zimmermann N, Wenk A, Kim U, et al. Functional and biochemical evaluation of platelet aspirin resistance after coronary artery bypass surgery. Circulation. 2003;108:542–7.

16. Michelson AD, Cattaneo M, Eikelboom JW, Gurbel P, Kottke-Marchant K, Kunicki TJ, Pulcinelli FM, Cerletti C, Rao AK. Platelet physiology subcommittee of the scientific and standardization committee of the international society on thrombosis and haemostasis; working group on aspirin resistance. Aspirin resistance: position paper of the working group on aspirin resistance. J Thromb Haemost. 2005;3:1309–11.

17. Haubelt H, Anders C, Vogt A, Hoerdt P, Seyfert UT, Hellstern P. Variables influencing platelet function analyzer-100 closure times in healthy individuals. Br J Haematol. 2005;130:759–67.

18. Hovens MM, Snoep JD, Eikenboom JC, et al. Prevalence of persistent platelet reactivity despite use of aspirin: a systematic review. Am Heart J. 2007;153:175–81.

19. Hurlen M, Seljeflot I, Arnesen H. The effect of different antithrombotic regimens on platelet aggregation after myocardial infarction. Scand Cardiovasc J. 1998;32:233–7.

20. Buchanan MR, Brister SJ. Individual variation in the effects of ASA on platelet function: implications for the use of ASA clinically. Can J Cardiol. 1995;11:221–7.

21. Buchanan MR, Schwartz L, Bourassa M, et al. Investigators. Results of the BRAT study—a pilot study investigating the possible significance of ASA nonresponsiveness on the benefits and risks of ASA on thrombosis in patients undergoing coronary artery bypass surgery. Can J Cardiol. 2000;16:1385–90.

22. Grotemeyer KH, Scharafinski HW, Husstedt IW. Two-year followup of aspirin responder and aspirin non responder. A pilot-study including 180 post-stroke patients. Thromb Res. 1993;71:397–403.

23. Gum PA, Kottke-Marchant K, Welsh PA, et al. A prospective, blinded determination of the natural history of aspirin resistance among stable patients with cardiovascular disease. J Am Coll Cardiol. 2003;41:961–5.

24. Gum PA, Kottke-Marchant K, Poggio ED, Sapp SK, Topol EJ, et al. Profile and prevalence of aspirin resistance in patients with cardiovascular disease. Am J Cardiol. 2001;88:230–5.

25. Eikelboom JW, Hirsh J, Weitz JI, et al. Aspirin-resistant thromboxane biosynthesis and the risk of myocardial infarction, stroke, or cardiovascular death in patients at high risk for cardiovascular events. Circulation. 2002;105:1650–5.

26. Eikelboom JW, Hankey GJ, Thom J, et al. Clopidogrel for high atherothrombotic risk and ischemic stabilization, management and avoidance (CHARISMA) investigators. Incomplete inhibition of thromboxane biosynthesis by acetylsalicylic acid: determinants and effect on cardiovascular risk. Circulation. 2008;118:1705–12.

27. Wang JC, Aucoin-Barry D, Manuelian D, et al. Incidence of aspirin nonresponsiveness using the Ultegra Rapid Platelet Function assay-ASA. Am J Cardiol. 2003;92:1492–4.

28. Chen WH, Lee PY, Ng W, et al. Aspirin resistance is associated with a high incidence of myonecrosis after non-urgent percutaneous coronary intervention despite clopidogrel pretreatment. J Am Coll Cardiol. 2004;43:1122–6.

29. Gonzalez-Conejero R, Rivera J, Corral J, et al. Biological assessment of aspirin efficacy on healthy individuals: heterogeneous response or aspirin failure? Stroke. 2005;36:276–80.

30. Tantry US, Bliden KP, Gurbel PA. Overestimation of platelet aspirin resistance detection by thrombelastograph platelet mapping and validation by conventional aggregometry using arachidonic acid stimulation. J Am Coll Cardiol. 2005;46:1705–9.

31. Schwartz KA, Schwartz DE, Ghosheh K, et al. Compliance as a critical consideration in patients who appear to be resistant to aspirin after healing of myocardial infarction. Am J Cardiol. 2005;95:973–5.

32. Gurbel PA, Bliden KP, DiChiara J, et al. Evaluation of dose-related effects of aspirin on platelet function: results from the aspirin-induced platelet effect (ASPECT) study. Circulation. 2007;115:3156–64.

33. Lordkipanidze M, Pharand C, Schampaert E, et al. A comparison of six major platelet function tests to determine the prevalence of aspirin resistance in patients with stable coronary artery disease. Eur Heart J. 2007;28:1702–8.

34. Faraday N, Becker DM, Yanek LR, et al. Relation between atherosclerosis risk factors and aspirin resistance in a primary prevention population. Am J Cardiol. 2006;98:774–9.

35. Frelinger III AL, Furman MI, Linden MD, et al. Residual arachidonic acid-induced platelet activation via an adenosine diphosphatedependent but cyclooxygenase-1– and cyclooxygenase-2–independent pathway: a 700-patient study of aspirin resistance. Circulation. 2006;113:2888–96.
36. Chen WH, Cheng X, Lee PY, et al. Aspirin resistance and adverse clinical events in patients with coronary artery disease. Am J Med. 2007;120:631–5.
37. Lev EI, Patel RT, Maresh KJ, et al. Aspirin and clopidogrel drug response in patients undergoing percutaneous coronary intervention: the role of dual drug resistance. J Am Coll Cardiol. 2006;47:27–33.
38. Marcucci R, Paniccia R, Antonucci E, et al. Usefulness of aspirin resistance after percutaneous coronary intervention for acute myocardial infarction in predicting one-year major adverse coronary events. Am J Cardiol. 2006;98:1156–9.
39. Gianetti J, Parri MS, Sbrana S, et al. Platelet activation predicts recurrent ischemic events after percutaneous coronary angioplasty: a 6 months prospective study. Thromb Res. 2006;118:487–93.
40. Foussas SG, Zairis MN, Patsourakos NG, et al. The impact of oral antiplatelet responsiveness on the long-term prognosis after coronary stenting. Am Heart J. 2007;154:676–81.
41. Malek LA, Spiewak M, Filipiak KJ, et al. Persistent platelet activation is related to very early cardiovascular events in patients with acute coronary syndromes. Kardiol Pol. 2007;65:40–5.
42. Borna C, Lazarowski E, van Heusden C, et al. Resistance to aspirin is increased by ST-elevation myocardial infarction and correlates with adenosine diphosphate levels. Thromb J. 2005;3:10.
43. DiChiara J, Bliden KP, Tantry US, et al. The effect of aspirin dosing on platelet function in diabetic and nondiabetic patients: an analysis from the aspirin-induced platelet effect (ASPECT) study. Diabetes. 2007;56:3014–9.
44. Jilma B, Fuchs I. Detecting aspirin resistance with the platelet function analyzer (PFA-100). Am J Cardiol. 2001;88:1348–9.
45. Addad F, Chakroun T, Elalamy I, Abderazek F, Chouchene S, Dridi Z, Gerotziafas GT, Hatmi M, Hassine M, Gamra H. Antiplatelet effect of once- or twice-daily aspirin dosage in stable coronary artery disease patients with diabetes. Int J Hematol. 2010;92:296–301.

46. Capodanno D, Patel A, Dharmashankar K, Ferreiro JL, Ueno M, Kodali M, Tomasello SD, Tello-Montoliu A, Kodali M, Capranzano P, Seecheran N, Darlington A, Montoliu AT, Desai Bass TA, Angiolillo DJ. Pharmacodynamic effects of different aspirin dosing regimens in type 2 diabetes mellitus patients with coronary artery disease. Circ Cardiovasc Interv. 2011;4:180–7.

47. Bliden KP, Tantry US, DiChiara J, Gurbel PA. Further ex vivo evidence supporting higher aspirin dosing in patients with coronary artery disease and diabetes. Circ Cardiovasc Interv. 2011;4:118–20.

48. Mueller MR, Salat A, Stangl P, et al. Variable platelet response to low-dose ASA and the risk of limb deterioration in patients submitted to peripheral arterial angioplasty. Thromb Haemost. 1997;78:1003–7.

49. Snoep JD, Hovens MM, Eikenboom JC, et al. Association of laboratory-defined aspirin resistance with a higher risk of recurrent cardiovascular events: a systematic review and meta-analysis. Arch Intern Med. 2007;167:1593–9.

50. Crescente M, Di Castelnuovo A, Iacoviello L, et al. Response variability to aspirin as assessed by the platelet function analyzer (PFA)-100. A systematic review. Thromb Haemost. 2008;99:14–26.

51. Reny JL, De Moerloose P, Dauzat M, et al. Use of the PFA-100 closure time to predict cardiovascular events in aspirin-treated cardiovascular patients: a systematic review and meta-analysis. J Thromb Haemost. 2008;6:444–50.

52. Breet NJ, van Werkum JW, Bouman HJ, Kelder JC, Harmsze AM, Hackeng CM, ten Berg JM. High on-treatment platelet reactivity to both aspirin and clopidogrel is associated with the highest risk of adverse events following percutaneous coronary intervention. Heart. 2011;97:983–90.

53. Dichiara J, Bliden KP, Tantry US, et al. Platelet function measured by VerifyNow identifies generalized high platelet reactivity in aspirin treated patients. Platelets. 2007;18:414–23.

54. Catella-Lawson F, Reilly MP, Kapoor SC, et al. Cyclooxygenase inhibitors and the antiplatelet effects of aspirin. N Engl J Med. 2001;345:1809–17.

55. Kurth T, Glynn RJ, Walker AM, et al. Inhibition of clinical benefits of aspirin on first myocardial infarction by nonsteroidal anti-inflammatory drugs. Circulation. 2003;108:1191–5.

56. Hennekens CH, Schneider WR, Hebert PR, Tantry US, Gurbel PA. Hypothesis formulation from subgroup analyses: nonadherence or nonsteroidal anti-inflammatory drug use explains the lack

of clinical benefit of aspirin on first myocardial infarction attributed to "aspirin resistance". Am Heart J. 2010;159:744–8.

57. Lev EI, Ramabadran RS, Guthikonda S, et al. Effect of ranitidine on the antiplatelet effects of aspirin in healthy human subjects. Am J Cardiol. 2007;99:124–8.

58. Goodman T, Ferro A, Sharma P. Pharmacogenetics of aspirin resistance: a comprehensive systematic review. Br J Clin Pharmacol. 2008;66:222–32.

59. Kuliczkowski W, Witkowski A, Polonski L, et al. Interindividual variability in the response to oral antiplatelet drugs: a position paper of the working group on antiplatelet drugs resistance appointed by the section of cardiovascular interventions of the polish cardiac society, endorsed by the working group on thrombosis of the European society of cardiology. Eur Heart J. 2009;30: 426–35.

60. Hagihara K, Kazui M, Kurihara A, Yoshiike M, Honda K, Okazaki O, Farid NA, Ikeda T. A possible mechanism for the differences in efficiency and variability of active metabolite formation from thienopyridine antiplatelet agents, prasugrel and clopidogrel. Drug Metab Dispos. 2009;37:2145–52.

61. Kazui M, Nishiya Y, Ishizuka T, Hagihara K, Farid NA, Okazaki O, Ikeda T, Kurihara A. Identification of the human cytochrome P450 enzymes involved in the two oxidative steps in the bioactivation of clopidogrel to its pharmacologically active metabolite. Drug Metab Dispos. 2010;38:92–9.

62. Savi P, Zachayus JL, Delesque-Touchard N, Labouret C, Hervé C, Uzabiaga MF, Pereillo JM, Culouscou JM, Bono F, Ferrara P, Herbert JM. The active metabolite of clopidogrel disrupts $P2Y_{12}$ receptor oligomers and partitions them out of lipid rafts. Proc Natl Acad Sci USA. 2006;103:11069–74.

63. Price MJ, Coleman JL, Steinhubl SR, Wong GB, Cannon CP, Teirstein PS. Onset and offset of platelet inhibition after high-dose clopidogrel loading and standard daily therapy measured by a point-of-care assay in healthy volunteers. Am J Cardiol. 2006;98: 681–4.

64. Gurbel PA, Bliden KP, Butler K, Tantry US, Gesheff T, Wei C, Teng R, Antonino MJ, Patil SB, Karunakaran A, Kereiakes DJ, Parris C, Purdy D, Wilson V, Ledley GS, Storey RF. Randomized double-blind assessment of the ONSET and OFFSET of the antiplatelet effects of ticagrelor versus clopidogrel in patients with stable coronary artery disease: the ONSET/OFFSET study. Circulation. 2009;120:2577–85.

65. Bonello L, Tantry US, Marcucci R, et al. Working group on high on-treatment platelet reactivity. Consensus and future directions on the definition of high on-treatment platelet reactivity to adenosine diphosphate. J Am Coll Cardiol. 2010;56:919–33.
66. French Registry of Acute ST-Elevation and Non-ST-Elevation Myocardial Infarction (FAST-MI) Investigators. Genetic determinants of response to clopidogrel and cardiovascular events. N Engl J Med. 2009;360:363–75.
67. Gurbel PA, Antonino MJ, Tantry US. Recent developments in clopidogrel pharmacology and their relation to clinical outcomes. Expert Opin Drug Metab Toxicol. 2009;5:989–1004.
68. Lau WC, Gurbel PA, Watkins PB, Neer CJ, Hopp AS, Carville DG, Guyer KE, Tait AR, Bates ER. Contribution of hepatic cytochrome P450 3A4 metabolic activity to the phenomenon of clopidogrel resistance. Circulation. 2004;109:166–71.
69. Lau WC, Welch TD, Shields T, et al. The effect of St John's Wort on the pharmacodynamic response of clopidogrel in hyporesponsive volunteers and patients: increased platelet inhibition by enhancement of CYP3A4 metabolic activity. J Cardiovasc Pharmacol. 2011;57:86–93.
70. Bliden KP, DiChiara J, Lookman L, Singla A, Antonino MJ, Baker BA, Bailey WL, Tantry US, Gurbel PA. The association of cigarette smoking with enhanced platelet inhibition by clopidogrel. J Am Coll Cardiol. 2008;52:531–3.
71. Berger JS, Bhatt DL, Steinhubl SR, Shao M, Steg PG, Montalescot G, Hacke W, Fox KA, Lincoff AM, Topol EJ, Berger PB. CHARISMA Investigators. Smoking, clopidogrel, and mortality in patients with established cardiovascular disease. Circulation. 2009;120:2337–44.
72. Desai NR, Mega JL, Jiang S, Cannon CP, Sabatine MS. Interaction between cigarette smoking and clinical benefit of clopidogrel. J Am Coll Cardiol. 2009;53:1273–8.
73. Gilard M, Arnaud B, Cornily JC, Le Gal G, Lacut K, Le Calvez G, Mansourati J, Mottier D, Abgrall JF, Boschat J. Influence of omeprazole on the antiplatelet action of clopidogrel associated with aspirin: the randomized, double-blind OCLA (Omeprazole CLopidogrel Aspirin) study. J Am Coll Cardiol. 2008;51:256–60.
74. Small DS, Farid NA, Payne CD, Weerakkody GJ, Li YG, Brandt JT, Salazar DE, Winters KJ. Effects of the proton pump inhibitor lansoprazole on the pharmacokinetics and pharmacodynamics of prasugrel and clopidogrel. J Clin Pharmacol. 2008;48:475–84.
75. Siller-Matula JM, Spiel AO, Lang IM, Kreiner G, Christ G, Jilma B. Effects of pantoprazole and esomeprazole on platelet inhibition by clopidogrel. Am Heart J. 2009;157:148.

76. Sibbing D, Morath T, Stegherr J, Braun S, Vogt W, Hadamitzky M, Schömig A, Kastrati A, von Beckerath N. Impact of proton pump inhibitors on the antiplatelet effects of clopidogrel. Thromb Haemost. 2009;10:714–9.
77. Ferreiro JL, Ueno M, Capodanno D, et al. Pharmacodynamic effects of concomitant versus staggered clopidogrel and omeprazole intake: results of a prospective randomized crossover study. Circ Cardiovasc Interv. 2010;3:436–41.
78. Angiolillo DJ, Gibson CM, Cheng S, et al. Differential effects of omeprazole and pantoprazole on the pharmacodynamics and pharmacokinetics of clopidogrel in healthy subjects: random-ized, placebo-controlled, crossover comparison studies. Clin Pharmacol Ther. 2011;89:65–74.
79. Gurbel PA, Bliden KP, Fort J, Zhang Y, Plachetka JR, Antonino M, Gesheff M, Tantry US. Pharmacodynamic evaluation of clopi-dogrel plus PA32540: the Spaced PA32540 With Clopidogrel Interaction Gauging (SPACING) study. Clin Pharmacol Ther. 2011;90:860–6.
80. Verstuyft C, Simon T, Kim RB. Personalized medicine and anti-platelet therapy: ready for prime time? Eur Heart J. 2009;30: 1943–63.
81. Angiolillo DJ, Fernandez-Ortiz A, Bernardo E, Ramírez C, Sabaté M, Jimenez-Quevedo P, Hernández R, Moreno R, Escaned J, Alfonso F, Bañuelos C, Costa MA, Bass TA, Macaya C. Platelet function profiles in patients with type 2 diabetes and coronary artery disease on combined aspirin and clopidogrel treatment. Diabetes. 2005;54:2430–5.
82. Angiolillo DJ, Fernández-Ortiz A, Bernardo E, Barrera Ramírez C, Sabaté M, Fernandez C, Hernández-Antolín R, Escaned J, Alfonso F, Macaya C. Platelet aggregation according to body mass index in patients undergoing coronary stenting: should clopidogrel loading-dose be weight adjusted? J Invasive Cardiol. 2004;16:169–74.
83. Sibbing D, von Beckerath O, Schömig A, Kastrati A, von Beckerath N. Platelet function in clopidogrel-treated patients with acute coronary syndrome. Blood Coagul Fibrinolysis. 2007;18:335–9.
84. Human Cytochrome0020P450 (CYP) Allele Nomenclature Committee. CYP2C19 allele nomenclature. 2011. http://www.cypalleles.ki.se/cyp2c19.htm. Accessed July 2011.
85. Scott SA, Sangkuhl K, Gardner EE, et al. Clinical pharmacoge-netics implementation consortium guidelines for cytochrome P450-2 C19 (CYP2C19) genotype and clopidogrel therapy. Clin Pharmacol Ther. 2011;90:328–32.

86. Gurbel PA, Shuldiner AR, Bliden KP, et al. The relation between CYP2C19 genotype and phenotype in stented patients on maintenance dual antiplatelet therapy. Am Heart J. 2011;161: 598–604.

87. Shuldiner AR, O'Connell JR, Bliden KP, et al. Association of cytochrome P450 2 C19 genotype with the antiplatelet effect and clinical efficacy of clopidogrel therapy. JAMA. 2009;302: 849–57.

88. Brandt JT, Close SL, Iturria SJ, Payne CD, Farid NA, Ernest 2nd CS, Lachno DR, Salazar D, Winters KJ. Common polymorphisms of CYP2C19 and CYP2C9 affect the pharmacokinetic and phar-macodynamic response to clopidogrel but not prasugrel. J Thromb Haemost. 2007;5:2429–36.

89. Mega JL, Close SL, Wiviott SD, Shen L, Hockett RD, Brandt JT, Walker JR, Antman EM, Macias W, Braunwald E, Sabatine MS. Cytochrome p-450 polymorphisms and response to clopidogrel. N Engl J Med. 2009;360:354–62.

90. Mega JL, Simon T, Collet JP, Anderson JL, et al. Reduced-function CYP2C19 genotype and risk of adverse clinical outcomes among patients treated with clopidogrel predomi-nantly for PCI: a meta-analysis. JAMA. 2010;304:1821–30.

91. Simon T, Verstuyft C, Mary-Krause M, Quteineh L, Drouet E, Méneveau N, Steg PG, Ferrières J, Danchin N, Becquemont L. French registry of acute ST-elevation and Non-ST-elevation myocardial infarction (FAST-MI) investigators. Genetic deter-minants of response to clopidogrel and cardiovascular events. N Engl J Med. 2009;360:363–75.

92. Pare G, Mehta SR, Yusuf S, et al. Effects of CYP2C19 genotype on outcomes of clopidogrel treatment. N Engl J Med. 2010;363: 1704–14.

93. Wallentin L, James S, Storey RF, Armstrong M, Barratt BJ, Horrow J, Husted S, Katus H, Steg PG, Shah SH. Becker RC Effect of CYP2C19 and ABCB1 single nucleotide polymor-phisms on outcomes of treatment with ticagrelor versus clopidogrel for acute coronary syndromes: A genetic substudy of the plato trial. Lancet. 2010;376:1320–8.

94. Price MJ, Tantry US, Gurbel PA. The influence of CYP2C19 polymorphisms on the pharmacokinetics, pharmacodynamics, and clinical effectiveness of P2Y(12) inhibitors. Rev Cardiovasc Med. 2011;12:1–12.

95. Bouman HJ, Schömig E, van Werkum JW, Velder J, Hackeng CM, Hirschhäuser C, Waldmann C, Schmalz HG, ten Berg JM, Taubert

D. Paraoxonase-1 is a major determinant of clopidogrel efficacy. Nat Med. 2011;17:110–6.

96. Price MJ, Murray SS, Angiolillo DJ et al. Primary results from genotype information and functional testing a prospective pharmacogenomic analysis of clopidogrel therapy. Presented at American College of Cardiology Meeting 2011 at New Orleans, USA; 2011.

97. Sibbing D, Koch W, Massberg S, et al. No association of paraoxonase-1 Q192R genotypes with platelet response to clopidogrel and risk of stent thrombosis after coronary stenting. Eur Heart J. 2011;32:1605–13.

98. Lewis JP, Fisch AS, Ryan K, O'Connell JR, et al. Paraoxonase 1 (PON1) Gene variants are not associated with clopidogrel response. Clin Pharmacol Ther. 2011. doi:10.1038/clpt.2011.194. [Epub ahead of print]

99. Gurbel PA, Bliden KP, Hiatt BL, O'Connor CM. Clopidogrel for coronary stenting: response variability, drug resistance, and the effect of pretreatment platelet reactivity. Circulation. 2003;107:2908–13.

100. Frelinger 3rd AL, Michelson AD, Wiviott SD, et al. Intrinsic platelet reactivity before P2Y12 blockade contributes to residual platelet reactivity despite high-level P2Y12 blockade by prasugrel or high-dose clopidogrel. Results from PRINCIPLE-TIMI 44. Thromb Haemost. 2011;106:219–26.

101. Michelson AD, Linden MD, Furman MI, et al. Evidence that pre-existent variability in platelet response to ADP accounts for 'clopidogrel resistance'. J Thromb Haemost. 2007;5:75–81.

102. Price MJ, Berger PB, Teirstein PS, et al. GRAVITAS Investigators. Standard- vs high-dose clopidogrel based on platelet function testing after percutaneous coronary intervention: the GRAVITAS randomized trial. JAMA. 2011;305:1097–105.

103. Campo G, Parrinello G, Ferraresi P, et al. Prospective evaluation of on-clopidogrel platelet reactivity over time in patients treated with percutaneous coronary intervention relationship with gene polymorphisms and clinical outcome. J Am Coll Cardiol. 2011;57:2474–83.

104. Järemo P, Lindahl TL, Fransson SG, Richter A. Individual variations of platelet inhibition after loading doses of clopidogrel. J Intern Med. 2002;252:233–8.

105. Bliden KP, DiChiara J, Tantry US, Bassi AK, Chaganti SK, Gurbel PA. Increased risk in patients with high platelet aggregation receiving chronic clopidogrel therapy undergoing percutaneous coronary intervention: is the current antiplatelet therapy adequate? J Am Coll Cardiol. 2007;49:657–66.

106. Gurbel PA, Bliden KP, Guyer K, Cho PW, Zaman KA, Kreutz RP, Bassi AK, Tantry US. Platelet reactivity in patients and recurrent

events post-stenting: results of the PREPARE POST-STENTING Study. J Am Coll Cardiol. 2005;46:1820–6.

107. Aleil B, Ravanat C, Cazenave JP, Rochoux G, Heitz A, Gachet C. Flow cytometric analysis of intraplatelet VASP phosphorylation for the detection of clopidogrel resistance in patients with ischemic cardiovascular diseases. J Thromb Haemost. 2005;3:85–92.

108. Barragan P, Bouvier JL, Roquebert PO, Macaluso G, Commeau P, Comet B, Lafont A, Camoin L, Walter U, Eigenthaler M. Resistance to thienopyridines: clinical detection of coronary stent thrombosis by monitoring of vasodilator-stimulated phosphoprotein phospho-rylation. Catheter Cardiovasc Interv. 2003;59:295–302.

109. Sibbing D, Braun S, Morath T, Mehilli J, Vogt W, Schömig A, Kastrati A, von Beckerath N. Platelet reactivity after clopidogrel treatment assessed with point-of-care analysis and early drug-elut-ing stent thrombosis. J Am Coll Cardiol. 2009;53:849–56.

110. Matetzky S, Shenkman B, Guetta V, et al. Clopidogrel resistance is associated with increased risk of recurrent atherothrombotic events in patients with acute myocardial infarction. Circulation. 2004;109:3171–5.

111. Gurbel PA, Bliden KP, Zaman KA, et al. Clopidogrel loading with eptifibatide to arrest the reactivity of platelets: results of the clopi-dogrel loading with eptifibatide to arrest the reactivity of platelets (CLEAR PLATELETS) study. Circulation. 2005;111:1153–9.

112. Gurbel PA, Bliden KP, Saucedo JF, et al. Bivalirudin and clopi-dogrel with and without eptifibatide for elective stenting: effects on platelet function, thrombelastographic indices and their relation to periprocedural infarction: results of the CLEAR PLATELETS-2 study. J Am Coll Cardiol. 2009;53:648–57.

113. Blindt R, Stellbrink K, de Taeye A, Müller R, Kiefer P, Yagmur E, Weber C, Kelm M, Hoffmann R. The significance of vasodilator-stimulated phosphoprotein for risk stratification of stent thrombosis. Thromb Haemost. 2007;98:1329–34.

114. Cuisset T, Frere C, Quilici J, et al. High post-treatment platelet reactivity is associated with a high incidence of myonecrosis after stenting for non-ST elevation acute coronary syndromes. Thromb Haemost. 2007;97:282–7.

115. Frere C, Cuisset T, Quilici J, Camoin L, Carvajal J, Morange PE, Lambert M, Juhan-Vague I, Bonnet JL, Alessi MC. ADP-induced platelet aggregation and platelet reactivity index VASP are good predictive markers for clinical outcomes in non-ST elevation acute coronary syndrome. Thromb Haemost. 2007;98:838–43.

116. Geisler T, Langer H, Wydymus M, et al. Low response to clopi-dogrel is associated with cardiovascular outcome after coronary stent implantation. Eur Heart J. 2006;27:2420–5.

117. Geisler T, Grass D, Bigalke B, Stellos K, Drosch T, Dietz K, Herdeg C, Gawaz M. The residual platelet aggregation after deployment of

intracoronary stent (PREDICT) score. J Thromb Haemost. 2008;6:54–61.

118. Hochholzer W, Trenk D, Bestehorn HP, et al. Impact of the degree of peri-interventional platelet inhibition after loading with clopidogrel on early clinical outcome of elective coronary stent placement. J Am Coll Cardiol. 2006;48:1742–50.

119. Price MJ, Endemann S, Gollapudi RR, et al. Prognostic significance of post-clopidogrel platelet reactivity assessed by a point-of-care assay on thrombotic events after drug-eluting stent implantation. Eur Heart J. 2008;29:992–1000.

120. Gurbel PA, Antonino MJ, Bliden KP, et al. Platelet reactivity to adenosine diphosphate and long-term ischemic event occurrence following percutaneous coronary intervention: a potential anti-platelet therapeutic target. Platelets. 2008;19:595–604.

121. Gurbel PA, Bliden KP, Samara W, et al. The clopidogrel resistance and stent thrombosis (CREST) study. J Am Coll Cardiol. 2005; 46:1827–32.

122. Buonamici P, Marcucci R, Miglironi A, et al. Impact of platelet reactivity after clopidogrel administration on drug-eluting stent thrombosis. J Am Coll Cardiol. 2007;49:2312–7.

123. Bonello L, Paganelli F, Arpin-Bornet M, et al. Vasodilator-stimulated phosphoprotein phosphorylation analysis prior to percutaneous coronary intervention for exclusion of postprocedural major adverse cardiovascular events. J Thromb Haemost. 2007;5:1630–6.

124. Cuisset T, Hamilos M, Sarma J, et al. Relation of low response to clopidogrel assessed with point-of-care assay to periprocedural myonecrosis in patients undergoing elective coronary stenting for stable angina pectoris. Am J Cardiol. 2008;101:1700–3.

125. Migliorini A, Valenti R, Marcucci R, Parodi G, Giuliani G, Buonamici P, Cerisano G, Carrabba N, Gensini GF, Abbate R, Antoniucci D. High residualplatelet reactivity after clopidogrel loading and long-term clinical outcomeafter drug-eluting stenting for unprotected left main coronary disease. Circulation. 2009;120: 2214–21.

126. Marcucci R, Gori AM, Paniccia R, et al. Cardiovascular death and nonfatal myocardial infarction in acute coronary syndrome patients receiving coronary stenting are predicted by residual platelet reactivity to ADP detected by a point-of-care assay: a 12-month follow- up. Circulation. 2009;119:237–342.

127. Patti G, Nusca A, Mangiacapra F, Gatto L, D'Ambrosio A, Di Sciascio G. Point-of-care measurement of clopidogrel responsiveness predicts clinical outcome in patients undergoing percutaneous coronary intervention results of the ARMYDA-PRO (antiplatelet therapy for reduction of MYocardial damage during angioplasty-platelet reactivity predicts outcome) study. J Am Coll Cardiol. 2008;52: 1128–33.

128. Cuisset T, Frere C, Quilici J, et al. Predictive values of post-treatment adenosinediphosphate-induced aggregation and vasodilator-stimulated phosphoprotein index for stent thrombosis after acute coronary syndrome in clopidogrel-treated patients. Am J Cardiol. 2009;104:1078–82.

129. Breet NJ, van Werkum JW, Bouman HJ, et al. Comparison of platelet function tests in predicting clinical outcome in patients undergoing coronary stent implantation. JAMA. 2010;303:754–62.

130. Samara WM, Bliden KP, Tantry US, Gurbel PA. The difference between clopidogrel responsiveness and posttreatment platelet reactivity. Thromb Res. 2005;115:89–94.

131. Tantry US, Bliden KP, Gurbel PA. What is the best measure of thrombotic risks–pretreatment platelet aggregation, clopidogrel responsiveness, or posttreatment platelet aggregation? Catheter Cardiovasc Interv. 2005;66:597–8.

132. Brar SS, Ten Berg J, Marcucci R, et al. Impact of platelet reactivity on clinical outcomes after percutaneous coronary intervention a collaborative meta-analysis of individual participant data. J Am Coll Cardiol. 2011;58:1945–54.

133. Stone GW. Assessment of dual antiplatelet therapy with drug-eluting stents a large-scale, prospective, multicenter registry examining the relationship between platelet responsiveness and stent Thrombosis after DES implantation. Presented at TCT 2011

134. Gurbel PA, Becker RC, Mann KG, Steinhubl SR, Michelson AD. Platelet function monitoring in patients with coronary artery disease. J Am Coll Cardiol. 2007;50:1822–34.

135. Yusuf S, Zhao F, Mehta SR, et al. The clopidogrel in unstable angina to prevent recurrent events TrialI. Effects of clopidogrel in addition to aspirin in patients with acute coronary syndromes without ST-segment elevation. N Engl J Med. 2001;345:494–502.

136. Wiviott SD, Braunwald E, McCabe CH, et al. TRITON-TIMI 38 investigators. Prasugrel versus clopidogrel in patients with acute coronary syndromes. N Engl J Med. 2007;357:2001–15.

137. Wallentin L, Becker RC, Budaj A, Cannon CP, Emanuelsson H, Held C, Horrow J, Husted S, James S, Katus H, Mahaffey KW, Scirica BM, Skene A, Steg PG, Storey RF, Harrington PLATO Investigators RA, Freij A, Thorsén M. Ticagrelor versus clopidogrel in patients with acute coronary syndromes. N Engl J Med. 2009;361:1045–57.

138. Sibbing D, Schulz S, Braun S, et al. Antiplatelet effects of clopidogrel and bleeding in patients undergoing coronary stent placement. J Thromb Haemost. 2010;8:250–6.

139. Gurbel PA, Bliden KP, Navickas IA, et al. Adenosine diphosphate-induced platelet-fibrin clot strength: a new thrombelastographic indicator of long-term poststenting ischemic events. Am Heart J. 2010;160:346–54.

140. Bracey L, Chen AW, Radovancevic R, et al. Clopidogrel and bleeding in patients undergoing elective coronary artery bypass grafting. J Thorac Cardiovasc Surg. 2004;128:425–31.
141. Mahla E, Suarez TA, Bliden KP, Rehak P, Metzler H, Sequeira AJ, Cho P, Sell J, Fan J, Antonino MJ, Tantry US, Gurbel PA. Platelet function measurement-based strategy to reduce bleeding and waiting time in clopidogrel-treated patients undergoing coronary artery bypass graft surgery: the timing based on platelet function strategy to reduce clopidogrel-associated bleeding related to CABG (TARGET-CABG) study. Circ Cardiovasc Interv. 2012;5:261–9.
142. Reece MJ, Klein AA, Salviz EA, et al. Near-patient platelet function testing in patients undergoing coronary artery surgery: a pilot study*. Anaesthesia. 2011;66:97–103.
143. Kwak YL, Kim JC, Choi YS, et al. Clopidogrel responsiveness regardless of the discontinuation date predicts increased blood loss and transfusion requirement after off-pump coronary artery bypass graft surgery. J Am Coll Cardiol. 2010;56:1994–2002.
144. Ranucci M, et al. Multiple electrode whole-blood aggregometry and bleeding in cardiac surgery patients receiving thienopyridines. Ann Thorac Surg. 2011;91:123–9.
145. Mokhtar OA, Lemesle G, Armero S, et al. Relationship between platelet reactivity inhibition and non-CABG related major bleeding in patients undergoing percutaneous coronary intervention. Thromb Res. 2010;126:e147–9.
146. Patti G, Pasceri V, Vizzi V, et al. Usefulness of platelet response to clopidogrel by point-of-care testing to predict bleeding outcomes in patients undergoing percutaneous coronary intervention (from the antiplatelet therapy for reduction of myocardial damage during angioplasty-bleeding study). Am J Cardiol. 2011;107:995–1000.
147. Cuisset T, Cayla G, Frere C, et al. Predictive value of post-treatment platelet reactivity for occurrence of post-discharge bleeding after non-ST elevation acute coronary syndrome. Shifting from antiplatelet resistance to bleeding risk assessment? Euro Interven. 2009;5:325–9.
148. Bonello L, Camoin-Jau L, Arques S, et al. Adjusted clopidogrel loading doses according to vasodilator-stimulated phosphoprotein phosphorylation index decrease rate of major adverse cardiovascular events in patients with clopidogrel resistance: a multicenter randomized prospective study. J Am Coll Cardiol. 2008;51:1404–11.
149. Bonello L, Camoin-Jau L, Armero S, Com O, Arques S, Burignat-Bonello C, Giacomoni MP, Bonello R, Collet F, Rossi P, Barragan P, Dignat-George F, Paganelli F. Tailored clopidogrel loading dose according to platelet reactivity monitoring to prevent acute and subacute stent thrombosis. Am J Cardiol. 2009;103:5–10.

150. Valgimigli M, Campo G, de Cesare N, et al. On behalf of tailoring treatment with tirofiban in patients showing resistance to aspirin and/or resistance to clopidogrel (3 T/2R) investigators. J Am Coll Cardiol. 2010;56:1447–55.

151. Cuisset T, Frere C, Quilici J, Morange PE, Mouret JP, Bali L, Moro PJ, Lambert M, Alessi MC, Bonnet JL. Glycoprotein IIb/IIIa inhibitors improve outcome after coronary stenting in clopidogrel nonresponders: a prospective, randomized study. JACC Cardiovasc Interv. 2008;1:649–53.

152. Angiolillo DJ, Shoemaker SB, Desai B, Yuan H, Charlton RK, Bernardo E, Zenni MM, Guzman LA, Bass TA, Costa MA. Randomized comparison of a high clopidogrel maintenance dose in patients with diabetes mellitus and coronary artery disease: results of the optimizing antiplatelet therapy in diabetes mellitus (OPTIMUS) study. Circulation. 2007;115:708–16.

153. von Beckerath N, Kastrati A, Wieczorek A, Pogatsa-Murray G, Sibbing D, Graf I, Schömig A. A double-blind, randomized study on platelet aggregation in patients treated with a daily dose of 150 or 75 mg of clopidogrel for 30 days. Eur Heart J. 2007;28:1814–9.

154. Angiolillo DJ, Costa MA, Shoemaker SB, Desai B, Bernardo E, Suzuki Y, Charlton RK, Zenni MM, Guzman LA, Bass TA. Functional effects of high clopidogrel maintenance dosing in patients with inadequate platelet inhibition on standard dose treatment. Am J Cardiol. 2008;101:440–5.

155. Matetzky S, Fefer P, Shenkman B, Varon D, Savion N, Hod H. Effectiveness of reloading to overcome clopidogrel nonresponsiveness in patients with acute myocardial infarction. Am J Cardiol. 2008;102:524–9.

156. Aleil B, Jacquemin L, De Poli F, Zaehringer M, Collet JP, Montalescot G, Cazenave JP, Dickele MC, Monassier JP, Gachet C. Clopidogrel 150 mg/day to overcome low responsiveness in patients undergoing elective percutaneous coronary intervention: results from the VASP-02 (vasodilator-stimulated phosphoprotein-02) randomized study. JACC Cardiovasc Interv. 2008;1:631–8.

157. Jeong YH, Lee SW, Choi BR, Kim IS, Seo MK, Kwak CH, Hwang JY, Park SW. Randomized comparison of adjunctive cilostazol versus high maintenance dose clopidogrel in patients with high post-treatment platelet reactivity: results of the ACCEL-RESISTANCE (adjunctive cilostazol versus high maintenance dose clopidogrel in patients with clopidogrel resistance) randomized study. J Am Coll Cardiol. 2009;53:1101–9.

158. Gurbel PA, Bliden KP, Antonino MJ, Stephens G, Gretler DD, Jurek MM, Pakyz RE, Shuldiner AR, Conley PB, Tantry US. The effect of elinogrel on high platelet reactivity during dual antiplatelet therapy and the relation to cyp 2c19*2 genotype: first experience in patients. J Thromb Haemost. 2010;8:43–53.

159. Gurbel PA, Bliden KP, Butler K, Antonino MJ, Wei C, Teng R, Rasmussen L, Storey RF, Nielsen T, Eikelboom J, Sabe-Affaki G, Husted S, Kereiakes DJ, Henderson D, Patel DV, Tantry US. Response to ticagrelor in clopidogrel Non-responders and Responders and the effect of switching therapies: the respond study. Circulation. 2010;121:1188–99.
160. Gurbel PA, Tantry US. An initial experiment with personalized antiplatelet therapy: the GRAVITAS trial. JAMA. 2011;305: 1136–7.
161. Price MJ, Angiolillo DJ, Teirstein PS, Lillie E, Manoukian SV, Berger PB, Tanguay JF, Cannon CP, Topol EJ. Platelet reactivity and cardiovascular outcomes after percutaneous coronary intervention: a time-dependent analysis of the gauging responsiveness with a VerifyNow P2Y12 assay: impact on thrombosis and safety (GRAVITAS) trial. Circulation. 2011;124:1132–7.
162. Trenk D, Stone GW, Gawaz M, Kastrati A, Angiolillo DJ, Müller U, Richardt G, Jakubowski JA, Neumann FJ. A randomized trial of prasugrel versus clopidogrel in patients with high platelet reactivity on clopidogrel after elective percutaneous coronary intervention with implantation of drug-eluting stents: results of the TRIGGER-PCI (Testing Platelet Reactivity In Patients Undergoing Elective Stent Placement on Clopidogrel to Guide Alternative Therapy With Prasugrel) study. J Am Coll Cardiol. 2012;59:2159–64.
163. Gurbel PA, Tantry US, Bliden KP, Jeong YH. Immunity to thrombotic events is achievable if we stop the guessing game: is this the major hidden message from GRAVITAS? Thromb Haemost. 2011;106:263–4.
164. Geisler T, Grass D, Bigalke B, et al. The residual platelet aggregation after deployment of intracoronary stent (PREDICT) score. J Thromb Haemost. 2008;6:54–61.
165. Levine GN, Bates ER, Blankenship JC, et al. 2011 ACCF/AHA/ SCAI guideline for percutaneous coronary intervention: a report of the American college of cardiology foundation/American heart association task force on practice guidelines and the society for cardiovascular angiography and interventions. Circulation. 2011;124: e574–651.
166. Wright RS, Anderson JL, Adams CD, Bridges CR, Casey Jr DE, Ettinger SM, Fesmire FM, Ganiats TG, Jneid H, Lincoff AM, Peterson ED, Philippides GJ, Theroux P, Wenger NK, Zidar JP, Jacobs AK. 2011 ACCF/AHA focused update of the guidelines for the management of patients with unstable angina/Non-ST-elevation myocardial infarction (updating the 2007 guideline): a report of the American college of cardiology foundation/American heart association task force on practice guidelines. Circulation. 2011;123: 2022–60.

167. Ferraris VA, Brown JR, Despotis GJ, Hammon JW, Reece TB, Saha SP, Song HK, Clough ER. Society of cardiovascular anesthesiologists special task force on blood transfusion, Shore-Lesserson LJ, Goodnough LT, Mazer CD, Shander A, Stafford-Smith M, Waters J. International Consortium for evidence based perfusion, Baker RA, Dickinson TA, FitzGerald DJ, Likosky DS, Shann KG. 2011 update to the society of thoracic surgeons and the society of cardiovascular anesthesiologists blood conservation clinical practice guidelines. Ann Thorac Surg. 2011;91:944–82.
168. Brilinta, FDA, drug insert. http://www1.astrazeneca-us.com/pi/brilinta.pdf. Accessed on 14 Aug 12.
169. Rinder CS, Bohnert J, Rinder HM, Mitchell J, Ault K, Hillman R. Platelet activation and aggregation during cardiopulmonary bypass. Anesthesiology. 1991;75:388–93.
170. Nuttall GA, Oliver WC, Santrach PJ, Bryant S, Dearani JA, Schaff HV, Ereth MH. Efficacy of a simple intraoperative transfusion algorithm for nonerythrocyte component utilization after cardiopulmonary bypass. Anesthesiology. 2001;94:773–81; discussion 5A-6A.
171. Shore-Lesserson L, et al. Thromboelastography-guided transfusion algorithm reduces transfusions in complex cardiac surgery. Anesth Analg. 1999;88:312–9.
172. Wasowicz M, McCluskey SA, Wijeysundera DN, Yau TM, Meinri M, Beattie WS, Karkouti K. The incremental value of thrombelastography for prediction of excessive blood loss after cardiac surgery: an observational study. Anesth Analg. 2010;111:331–8.
173. Chin CT, Roe MT, Fox KA, Prabhakaran D, et al. TRILOGY ACS Steering Committee. Study design and rationale of a comparison of prasugrel and clopidogrel in medically managed patients with unstable angina/non-ST-segment elevation myocardial infarction: the Targeted platelet inhibition to clarify the optimal strategy to medically manage acute coronary syndromes (TRILOGY ACS) trial. Am Heart J. 2010;160:16–22. e1.
174. Hamm CW, Bassand JP, Agewall S, et al. ESC guidelines for the management of acute coronary syndromes in patients presenting without persistent ST-segment elevation: the task force for the management of acute coronary syndromes (ACS) in patients presenting without persistent ST-segment elevation of the European society of cardiology (ESC). Eur Heart J. 2011;2011(32):2999–3054.

Chapter 3
Anticoagulant Drugs: Current and Novel

Daniel M. Witt and Nathan P. Clark

Introduction

The injectable anticoagulant unfractionated heparin (UFH), identified nearly a century ago by researchers at Johns Hopkins Medical School, was first used in humans in 1937 and still enjoys widespread use today [1]. During The Great Depression, financially strapped farmers in the Canadian prairies and Northern Plains of the United States were forced to feed their livestock moldy sweet clover hay resulting in the death from internal bleeding of previously healthy animals [1]. The investigation into the cause of this devastating blow to the farmers' livelihoods eventually culminated in the discovery of the world's most widely used oral anticoagulant, warfarin [1]. Decades elapsed before the next advance in

D.M. Witt, PharmD, FCCP, BCPS (✉)
Department of Pharmacy, Clinical Pharmacy Research & Applied
Pharmacogenomics, Kaiser Permanente Colorado,
16601 East Centretech Parkway, Aurora, CO 80011, USA
e-mail: dan.m.witt@kp.org

N.P. Clark, PharmD, BCPS, CACP
Department of Pharmacy, Clinical Pharmacy Anticoagulation & Anemia
Service, Kaiser Permanente Colorado, 16601 East Centretech Parkway,
Aurora, CO 80011, USA
e-mail: nathan.clark@kp.org

A. Ferro, D.A. Garcia (eds.), *Antiplatelet and Anticoagulation*   113
Therapy, Current Cardiovascular Therapy,
DOI 10.1007/978-1-4471-4297-3_3,
© Springer-Verlag London 2013

anticoagulation therapy, low-molecular-weight heparin (LMWH) was introduced into widespread use in the mid 1990s. Since then, several new anticoagulants including argatroban, bivalirudin, lepirudin, fondaparinux, dabigatran, and rivaroxaban have become available, with numerous others likely to be marketed in the near future.

Understanding the basic pharmacologic and pharmacokinetic properties of available anticoagulants is necessary in order to select the agent that will have the greatest likelihood of producing favorable clinical outcomes. This chapter will review, compare, and contrast these properties for both traditional and new anticoagulants with emphasis on associated clinical outcomes.

Attributes of the Ideal Anticoagulant

Various authorities have offered opinions on the attributes of the 'ideal' anticoagulant. Common elements include predictable pharmacokinetics and pharmacodynamics, rapid onset and offset of effect, minimal adverse effects, low drug-drug or drug-food interaction potential, a wide therapeutic index, no need for routine coagulation test monitoring, oral administration, availability of an antidote for reversal of anticoagulant effect, and once-daily dosing [2]. Unfortunately, none of the available anticoagulants, including those most recently introduced for clinical use, satisfies all of these criteria. In fact, the introduction of new anticoagulants has resulted in thoughtful reevaluation of whether some of these criteria really do define the ideal agent after all.

For example, rapid offset of effect may be ideal when interrupting therapy for an invasive procedure. However, it may also increase the risk of therapeutic failure associated with missed doses and transitions between different agents (e.g. switching from rivaroxaban to warfarin) [3]. Not needing to routinely monitor coagulation tests is generally considered ideal, but the ability to accurately assess the intensity of anticoagulant effect with a widely available laboratory test is desirable in certain clinical situations. The availability of alternatives to UFH and warfarin is certainly an important therapeutic advance, but one that makes knowledge of the pharmacokinetic and pharmacodynamic properties of anticoagulants more important than ever.

Hemostasis Basics

A brief overview of the physiology underlying normal coagulation of blood is provided as background for understanding the mechanisms of action for anticoagulants discussed hereafter. Hemostasis occurs in a series of distinct but overlapping steps (see Fig. 3.1) [4]. Normally, endothelial cells lining the interior surface of blood vessels maintain blood flow by physically separating extra vascular collagen and tissue factor from platelets, but vascular injury allows contact with the extra vascular space, ultimately initiating the process of fibrin formation. Initially, tissue factor bearing cells produce small (picomolar) amounts of thrombin via the factor VIIa/tissue factor and the factor Xa/Va complexes (traditionally referred to as the 'extrinsic' coagulation pathway) [5]. This initial thrombin generation is insufficient to arrest bleeding, but amplifies the hemostatic process by activating platelets at the site of vascular injury [4]. This facilitates the activation of cofactors V and VIII and factor XI on platelet surfaces in preparation for large-scale thrombin production. Much of what has traditionally been termed the 'intrinsic' coagulation pathway (namely factor XIa, the factor IXa/VIIIa complex and the factor Xa/Va complex) occurs during this process on negatively charged phospholipid surfaces of activated platelets (see Fig. 3.1). Thus, the intrinsic and extrinsic pathways cannot function as independent, redundant pathways in vivo, but are both required for physiologic hemostasis operating on different cell surfaces and playing unique roles [4].

Fibrin clot forms through the thrombin-mediated conversion of soluble fibrinogen to form fibrin monomers that eventually reach a critical concentration where they precipitate and polymerize to form fibrin strands. Following activation by thrombin, factor XIIIa covalently binds these strands to one

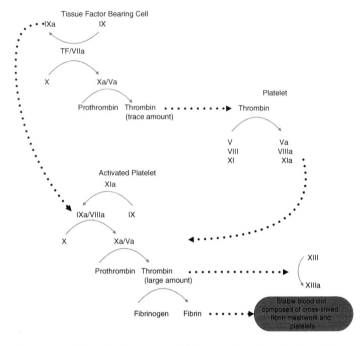

FIGURE 3.1 Physiologic process of fibrin clot formation (Adapted from Monroe and Hoffman [4], Mann et al. [5], and Crawley et al. [6])

another, forming an extensive meshwork that surrounds and encases aggregated platelets to form a stabilized clot that seals the site of vascular injury and arrests bleeding [6]. When this expanding meshwork of platelets and fibrin 'paves over' the initiation site, activated factors are unable to diffuse through the overlying layer of clot, and coagulation is effectively terminated [4].

The intact endothelium adjacent to the damaged tissue actively secretes thrombomodulin which modulates thrombin activity by converting protein C to its active form (activated protein C [aPC]) [6]. When joined with its cofactor protein S, aPC attenuates clot formation by inactivating factors Va and VIIIa. Antithrombin is a circulating protein that inhibits thrombin and factor Xa. Heparan sulfate, a heparin-like compound secreted by endothelial cells, exponentially accelerates antithrombin activity. When these endogenous self-regulatory mechanisms are intact, formation of fibrin clot is limited to the site of tissue injury. However, disruptions in this system of self-regulation can result in pathologic thrombosis [7].

Mechanisms of Action — Available Anticoagulants

Thrombin (IIa) plays a central role in controlling clot formation, both accelerating and attenuating the process [6]. Several anticoagulants exert their anticoagulant effect by interfering with thrombin either indirectly (UFH, LMWH, warfarin) or directly (dabigatran, bivalirudin, argatroban, and lepirudin). Thrombin is activated by factor Xa which is inhibited indirectly by UFH, LMWH, fondaparinux, and warfarin, and directly by rivaroxaban and apixaban. Warfarin also reduces the activity of factors VIIa, IXa and proteins C and S, while UFH also inhibits the activity of factors IXa, XIa and XIIa [8].

The mechanisms of action for available anticoagulants are summarized in Table 3.1. Unfractionated heparin, LMWH, and fondaparinux are indirect coagulation inhibitors that rely upon endogenous antithrombin to exert their anticoagulant effect. Warfarin and other vitamin K antagonists are also considered indirect coagulation inhibitors because their anticoagulant effect is mediated through enzymes responsible for the cyclic conversion of vitamin K in the liver. Indirect coagulation inhibitors are not active against thrombin or factor Xa within a formed clot or bound to surfaces. Fibrin-bound thrombin that remains active continues to promote clot growth [2]. Therefore, agents like direct thrombin inhibitors and direct Xa inhibitors capable of inhibiting clot-bound thrombin or factor Xa, respectively, may more effectively inhibit clot formation, but whether this translates into clinically superior anticoagulation remains to be conclusively demonstrated. Selective inhibition of factor Xa may provide more efficient control over fibrin generation by preserving thrombin's regulatory functions

TABLE 3.1 Mechanism of action of anticoagulant drugs

Vitamin K antagonists, warfarin, phenprocoumon, acenocoumarol	Inhibition of the enzymes responsible for the cyclic conversion of vitamin K in the liver which is required for the biologic activity of the vitamin K-dependent coagulation proteins, namely factors II (prothrombin), VII, IX, and X, as well as the endogenous anticoagulant proteins C and S—no direct effect on previously circulating clotting factors or previously formed thrombus. Not active against fibrin bound thrombin
Unfractionated heparin	Inhibits the activity of several clotting factors including IXa, Xa, XIIa, and thrombin through a specific pentasaccharide sequence that binds to antithrombin; the UFH–antithrombin complex inhibits thrombin and activated factor X 100–1,000 times more potently than antithrombin alone. Also inhibits the thrombin-induced activation of factors V and VIII. Thrombin and Xa are the most sensitive to inhibition by the UFH–antithrombin complex. Not active against fibrin bound thrombin
Low-molecular-weight heparin, enoxaparin, dalteparin, tinzaparin	Like UFH, the LMWHs enhance and accelerate the activity of antithrombin through binding to a specific pentasaccharide sequence; the principal difference in the pharmacologic activity of the LMWHs and UFH is their relative inhibition of factor Xa and thrombin; LMWHs have limited activity against thrombin (ratio of antifactor Xa-to-IIa activity varies between 4:1 and 2:1)—UFH has an antifactor Xa-to-IIa activity ratio of 1:1. Because they exhibit less binding to plasma proteins and endothelial cells, LMWH have more consistent bioavailability than UFH. LMWH are not active against fibrin bound thrombin

Pentasaccharide, fondaparinux	Similar to UFH and the LMWHs; through interaction with antithrombin; unlike UFH and LMWH, no direct effect on thrombin activity. Does not induce the formation of anti-heparin-PF4 antibodies; virtually no risk for HIT
Direct factor Xa inhibitors, rivaroxaban, apixaban	Competitive inhibition of free and fibrin-bound factor Xa; do not require antithrombin to inhibit factor Xa
Direct thrombin inhibitors, dabigatran, lepirudin, bivalirudin, argatroban	Interferes irreversibly (lepirudin) or reversibly (dabigatran, bivalirudin, argatroban) with the active site of both free and fibrin-bound thrombin

in the control of hemostasis, but this has also not translated into a definitive clinical advantage [9].

Clinical Implications of Anticoagulant Drug Pharmacokinetic Properties

Absorption and Distribution

Drugs given intravenously directly enter the bloodstream. Oral administration requires a drug to pass through the gut wall to enter the blood stream. Likewise, drugs administered subcutaneously must be absorbed into the bloodstream from the injection site. These latter processes are affected by many factors such as product formulation, stability during exposure to acid and enzymes, motility of the gut, presence of food in the stomach, and lipid solubility. Bioavailability or proportion of administered drug that reaches the plasma, of orally and subcutaneously administered drugs varies with different drugs and also from patient to patient, whereas the bioavailability of intravenously administered drugs is 100 %. Bioavailability of intramuscular injection is often nearly complete; however, anticoagulants are not administered by this route due to the risk of hematoma.

Following absorption into the bloodstream, drugs distribute among assorted proteins and tissues. Some drugs are retained primarily in the vascular compartment, others to the extra vascular fluid, while others distribute throughout the total body water or concentrate in certain tissues. In general terms, drugs that are highly protein bound or have high molecular weight are retained in the circulation, highly ionized drugs are confined to extra cellular fluid, and lipid-soluble drugs enter cells. Volume of distribution is a parameter used to describe the apparent volume into which a given drug is distributed. Volumes of distribution greater than 15 L indicate total body water distribution or concentration in tissues. Pharmacokinetic parameters relating to distribution for various anticoagulant drugs are summarized in Table 3.2.

TABLE 3.2 Absorption and distribution parameters of anticoagulant drugs [3, 10, 20, 22–25, 29, 31, 38, 39, 41, 50]

Drug	Route of administration	Onset of effect	Volume of distribution[a] (L)	Plasma protein binding
Unfractionated heparin	IV, SC	2–4 h (SC)	4.9	Extensive
Low-molecular-weight heparins				
Dalteparin	IV, SC	3–5 h (SC)	3.5	Less than UFH
Enoxaparin	IV, SC	3–5 h (SC)	4.3	Less than UFH
Tinzaparin	SC	3–5 h	3.1–5	Less than UFH
Pentasaccharide				
Fondaparinux	SC	2–3 h	7–11	Minimal
Direct factor Xa inhibitors				
Apixaban	Oral	3–4 h	22	87 %
Rivaroxaban	Oral	2–4 h	50	92–95 %
Direct thrombin inhibitors				
Argatroban	IV		12.2	
Bivalirudin	IV		21	
Dabigatran	Oral	1–2 h	50–70	35 %
Lepirudin	IV, SC		17–23	
Vitamin K antagonists				
Warfarin	Oral, IV	3–5d	9.8	99 %
Acenocoumarol	Oral	3–5d	11.2–23.8	99 %
Phenprocoumon	Oral	3–5d	6.5	99 %

h hours, *L* liters, *IV* intravenous, *SC* subcutaneous, *UFH* unfractionated heparin, *d* days
[a]Calculated for 70 kg male where reported in package insert as L/kg

Unfractionated and Low-Molecular-Weight Heparin

Unfractionated heparin is a heterogeneous mixture of negatively charged glycosaminoglycans of varying sizes. Unfractionated heparin has little or no oral bioavailability and therefore must be administered via intravenous or subcutaneous injection [10]. Unfractionated heparin interacts with multiple proteins and cellular membranes which influence its subcutaneous absorption, anticoagulant activity, and adverse effect profile [11]. These cellular and protein interactions can reduce the activity of UFH and thus result in an unpredictable anticoagulant effect (assessed in clinical practice by measuring the activated partial thromboplastin time (aPTT) or anti-factor Xa activity) [10]. When UFH is administered subcutaneously, higher doses are required to compensate for reduced bioavailability arising from binding interactions at the injection site [10]. Unfractionated heparin impairs osteoblast formation and activates osteoclasts; these actions can result in osteopenia [10]. Heparin-inducted thrombocytopenia, a potentially life-threatening complication of UFH therapy, is attributable to antibodies directed at complexes formed by platelet factor 4 (PF4) binding to UFH [12].

Commercially available LMWH are produced from porcine mucosal heparin using chemical or enzymatic depolarization [10]. Although the process for each product is unique, the resulting consistency of smaller heparin molecules avoids or minimizes many of the UFH interactions with plasma proteins and cellular membranes. Like UFH, LMWH has little or no oral bioavailability. Protein binding is low, resulting in a more predictable dose–response and greater subcutaneous bioavailability (90 %) than UFH [10]. Decreased binding to platelets results in a lower risk of HIT, particularly postoperatively [12]. Medical patients with venous thromboembolism have a low risk of HIT regardless of heparin preparation [13]. Although platelet binding is reduced, LMWH can still form complexes with PF4 capable of binding HIT antibodies. Because of this cross-reactivity, LMWH should be avoided in patients with HIT antibodies [10].

Reduction in bone mineral density has been reported with LMWH [14] but is the effect is less prominent than that seen with UFH [10].

Low-molecular-weight heparins are dosed according to weight and renal function. Unlike UFH, routine laboratory monitoring of LMWH is unnecessary [10]. Because LMWH are largely concentrated in plasma, it has been debated whether total body weight, lean body weight or ideal body weight, should be used for dose determination. While some have suggested there should be a maximal dose used for very obese patients, the balance of evidence and opinion suggests dose capping is not warranted and total body weight should be used to calculate LMWH doses [15, 16].

Pentasaccharide

Fondaparinux is a synthetic analog of the antithrombin-binding pentasaccharide sequence found in UFH and LMWH [10]. Fondaparinux is not absorbed orally but is rapidly and completely absorbed following subcutaneous injection [10]. Fondaparinux is highly bound to antithrombin but has little affinity for other plasma proteins or platelets [17]. As a result of limited platelet interaction, fondaparinux is commonly used for prevention or treatment of venous thromboembolism where a history of HIT precludes the use of UFH or LWMH. Although fondaparinux is not licensed for the treatment of HIT (with or without thrombosis), indirect evidence suggests that it would be a safe and effective treatment in this setting [18].

Direct Factor Xa Inhibitors

Rivaroxaban's oral absorption is dose dependent. Lower doses (10 mg) have a bioavailability of 80–100 % and are unaffected by food. Higher doses (15–20 mg) have reduced bioavailability (~66 % in the fasted state) that is increased by administration with food. For this reason, it is recommended that doses of 15 and 20 mg be taken with food [3]. Rivaroxaban is a substrate of the P-glycoprotein (P-gp) efflux transporter [3]. P-glycoprotein is expressed in multiple organs that influence drug disposition such as small intestine, blood–brain barrier, kidney, and liver. Drugs that induce intestinal P-gp activity can reduce bioavailability of orally administered drugs and decrease therapeutic effect. Conversely, P-gp inhibition can lead to increased bioavailability, and an increased risk of toxicity [19]. Drugs that affect both P-gp and metabolizing enzymes have the potential to result in clinically significant drug interactions with rivaroxaban [3]. This topic will be addressed later in the section on metabolism and elimination. Apixaban is rapidly absorbed after oral administration with an absolute bioavailability of around 50 % at usual doses. Food does not appear to affect apixaban bioavailability [20]. Apixaban is also a P-gp substrate and subject to interactions with drugs that affect both P-gp and metabolizing enzymes (addressed later in metabolism and elimination section) [20].

Rivaroxaban and apixaban both selectively bind to factor Xa and have similar distribution properties [3, 21]. Binding to plasma protein ranges from 87 % for apixaban to 95 % for rivaroxaban, with rivaroxaban binding primarily to albumin [3, 20]. The volume of distribution for both drugs indicates distribution to tissue [3, 20].

Direct Thrombin Inhibitors

Dabigatran is the only direct thrombin inhibitor that is absorbed orally. Commercially available capsules are formulated as dabigatran etexilate mesylate and absorbed as the prodrug dabigatran etexilate which is hydrolyzed to form active dabigatran. Bioavailability is only 3–7 %, and is not affected by food [22]. Dabigatran is a P-gp substrate and drugs that inhibit and induce P-gp can increase and decrease dabigatran exposure, respectively [22]. The use of dabigatran in combination with P-gp inducers (e.g. rifampin) should be avoided [22].

Argatroban, bivalirudin, and lepirudin have little or no oral bioavailability and are labeled for use by intravenous administration only [23–25]. However, lepirudin has been administered successfully subcutaneously [26–28]. Drugs known to increase the risk of bleeding due to antiplatelet or anticoagulant effects increase the risk of bleeding when used in combination with argatroban, bivalirudin, and lepirudin [23–25].

The volume of distribution among direct thrombin inhibitors ranges from 0.17 L/kg for argatroban to 0.9 L/kg for dabigatran [22, 23]. Dabigatran is a small molecule; only 35 % is bound to plasma proteins, allowing it to be removed by dialysis if needed.

Vitamin K Antagonists

Warfarin is rapidly and completely absorbed following oral administration and may be taken with or without food [29]. Absorption of warfarin from the gastrointestinal tract can be impaired by bile acid sequestrants, such as cholestyramine or colestipol [30]. Although warfarin is rapidly absorbed, therapeutic anticoagulation requires the elimination of vitamin K-dependent clotting factors (II, VII, IX and X) synthesized prior to warfarin ingestion. Because of the half-lives of these proteases, the anticoagulant effect of warfarin is usually not obtained for approximately 5 days after initiation [31]. Therefore, in the setting of acute thrombosis, warfarin is usually initiated in conjunction with a more rapidly acting anticoagulant (e.g. UFH, LMWH, fondaparinux) for at least 5 days [31].

Vitamin K antagonists are highly protein bound. Warfarin is 99 % bound to plasma proteins, mostly albumin [31]. Other drugs that are highly bound to albumin may compete for protein binding, displacing warfarin and increasing free warfarin concentrations in plasma. While displacement drug interactions may cause an increase in warfarin's hypoprothrombinemic effect as measured by the INR, the effect is usually transient as free warfarin is readily metabolized [30]. Drugs that both displace warfarin from plasma proteins and inhibit warfarin metabolism (e.g. co-trimoxazole) have high potential to cause excessive anticoagulation [32]. Warfarin crosses the placenta and fetal warfarin serum concentrations approach that of the mother. Warfarin is a known teratogen and increases the risk of both fetal and maternal hemorrhage during labor and delivery [29]. For this reason, warfarin is generally avoided during pregnancy and women of childbearing potential should take precautions not to become pregnant during warfarin therapy [29]. Active warfarin is not found in breast milk and is generally considered acceptable for breast feeding mothers [33].

Metabolism and Elimination

Drugs are metabolized mainly to hasten their elimination from the body. The liver is the main organ responsible for drug metabolism, most commonly via an important class of enzymes called cytochrome p450 mixed function oxidases. Synthesis of cytochrome p450 enzymes can be induced by repeated administration of some drugs resulting in increased clearance of p450 substrates. Conversely, some drugs can inhibit p450 enzyme activity resulting in reduced metabolism and enhanced (or prolonged) effect of p450 substrates [34]. Most drugs are ultimately eliminated from the body via the kidneys, but some drugs are concentrated in the bile and excreted into the intestine where they can be eliminated in the feces or reabsorbed. This latter process is termed enterohepatic circulation and increases the residence time of affected drugs. Anticoagulant drug pharmacokinetic parameters relating to metabolism and elimination are summarized in Table 3.3.

Heparin and Low-Molecular-Weight Heparins

Unfractionated heparin is cleared by both a rapid, saturable mechanism as well as a slower first-order process [10]. Larger UFH molecules are more rapidly cleared than smaller fractions. Receptors on endothelial cells and macrophages bind UFH and facilitate clearance through depolymerization. The

TABLE 3.3 Metabolism and elimination parameters of anticoagulant drugs [3, 10, 20, 22–25, 29, 31, 38, 39, 41, 50]

Drug	Primary	Secondary	Half – life
Unfractionated heparin	Reticulo-endothelial depolymerization	Renal excretion	0.5–2 h (dose dependent)
Low-molecular-weight heparins			
Dalteparin	Renal excretion		3–5 h
Enoxaparin	Renal excretion		4.5 h
Tinzaparin	Renal excretion		3–4 h
Pentasaccharide			
Fondaparinux	Renal excretion		17–21 h
Direct factor Xa inhibitors			
Apixaban	Renal excretion	Liver metabolism (CYP 3A4)	8–13 h
Rivaroxaban	Renal excretion	Liver metabolism (CYP 3A4)	5–9 h
Direct thrombin inhibitors			
Argatroban	Liver metabolism		0.5–0.85 h
Bivalirudin	Renal metabolism (proteolytic cleavage)		
Dabigatran	Renal excretion	Liver metabolism (CYP 3A4)	12–17 h
Lepirudin	Renal excretion		1.3 h
Vitamin K antagonists			
Warfarin	Liver metabolism (CYP450 2C9)	Liver metabolism (CYP 3A4, 2C19, 1A2)	20–60 h
Acenocoumoral	Liver metabolism (CYP450 2C9)		8–11 h
Phenprocoumon	Liver metabolism (CYP 2C9, 3A4)	Renal excretion, bile excretion	96–144 h

h hours

slower, nonsaturable mechanism relies on renal elimination. As a result of this bimodal elimination process, larger UFH doses produce longer half-lives and greater bioavailability [10]. Although UFH elimination is complex, its short half life (60–90 min) and non-renal elimination constitute two of the few remaining advantages of UFH over LMWH. Clinically, UFH is often preferred in situations where anticoagulation may need to be reversed quickly (e.g. surgery), or in patients with renal insufficiency.

In clinical situations where UFH must be reversed urgently or where the effect of UFH is likely to persist for an extended period, such as after a large subcutaneous dose, an antidote is available. Protamine sulfate is a basic protein that complexes with UFH to rapidly reverse its anticoagulant effect. One milligram of protamine sulfate inactivates approximately 100 Units of UFH [10]. Typical doses of range from 30 to 50 mg depending on the degree of UFH exposure. Protamine sulfate retains the ability to neutralize the anti-factor IIa activity of LMWH as well, but its effectiveness in arresting bleeding in patients receiving LMWH remains to be elucidated [10].

Elimination of LMWH is primarily renal. Unlike UFH, clearance of LMWH is independent of dose [10]. The potential for LMWH accumulation increases with decreasing renal function, particularly when creatinine clearance (CrCL) is less than 30 mL/min [35, 36]. There have been several reports of LWMH accumulation with varying degrees of renal insufficiency, but the exact CrCL rate where the risk of LMWH accumulation begins is likely product-specific [35, 37]. Commercially available LMWH products have unique pharmacokinetic parameters including half-life and proportion of total drug clearance as renal elimination. Tinzaparin, which is relatively larger, on average, than either dalteparin or enoxaparin, relies less on renal elimination [16]. Enoxaparin, the LMWH which relies most on renal elimination, provides specific dose guidelines in the setting of CrCL less than 30 mL/min in its prescribing information [38]. These recommendations are based upon an unpublished proprietary pharmacokinetic analysis [38]. Clinical trial data evaluating the safety and efficacy of recommended renally-adjusted enox-aparin doses are lacking. Dalteparin use is recommended 'with caution' when CrCL is less than 30 mL/min [39].

Chronic kidney disease is a prevalent comorbidity among patients requiring antithrombotic therapy and this presents challenges for prescribers of LMWH. Monitoring the anticoagulant response in patients with renal insufficiency receiving LMWH is often recommended. However, coagulation monitoring for LMWH suffers from lack of standardization [40]. Low-molecular-weight heparins vary in their activity as measured by the aPTT rendering this test useless for monitoring LMWH [10]. The most common test used to monitor the anticoagulant effect of LMWH is the anti-factor Xa assay. However, the evidence correlating elevated anti-factor Xa activity with bleeding risk or low activity with treatment failure is limited. Thus, therapeutic anti-factor Xa ranges for LMWH have yet to be definitely established or tested. Commercially available LMWH have unique anti-factor Xa versus anti-factor IIa profiles, yet clinical laboratories typically report only one reference range, or set of ranges for therapeutic, intermediate, or prophylactic LMWH anti-factor Xa levels that are not drug-specific. The relevance and reliability of LMWH anti-factor Xa monitoring continues to be debated [16]. Overall, lack of need for routine monitoring is a major advantage of LMWH compared to UFH. However, in the setting of renal insufficiency, or in patient populations under-represented in clinical trials (e.g. obesity, pregnancy), the lack of a standardized method to monitor the anticoagulant effect of LMWH is a disadvantage.

Pentasaccharide

Fondaparinux relies completely on renal elimination, and is contraindicated in patients with CrCL <30 mL/min [41]. Relative to LMWH, fondaparinux has a long half-life (~4 h vs. 17–21 h, respectively) [41]. The longer half-life is convenient for once daily dosing in management or prevention of venous thromboembolism, but also presents challenges.

Because of rapid onset and offset of effect, LMWH is frequently used as cross-coverage when warfarin therapy must be interrupted for invasive procedures, a process known as "bridge" therapy. The long half-life and slow offset of fondaparinux limit its utility in this setting, particularly when used preoperatively. Management of postoperative bleeding is complicated by a long half-life and lack of a known antidote to reverse anticoagulant effect. Thus, fondaparinux has a limited role in bridge therapy.

Direct Factor Xa Inhibitors

Rivaroxaban and apixaban are both cleared by a combination of hepatic metabolism and renal elimination [3, 21]. Just over half of an orally administered rivaroxaban dose is metabolized, primarily by CYP 3A4/5 and CYP 2J2 [3]. Approximately 25 % of apixaban is metabolized, mainly by CYP 3A4/5 [20]. As mentioned previously, both rivaroxaban and apixaban are substrates of the P-gp efflux transporter [3, 20]. Concomitant use of drugs that both inhibit P-gp and are strong inhibitors of CYP 3A4 (e.g. ketoconazole, itraconazole, voriconazole, ritonavir, conivaptan, clarithromycin) can result in significant increases in rivaroxaban or apixaban exposure and heightened bleeding risk [3, 20]. Conversely, concomitant use of drugs that are combined P-gp and strong CYP 3A4 inducers (e.g. carbamazepine, phenytoin, rifampicin, St. John's wort) may reduce exposure to rivaroxaban or apixaban and decrease efficacy [3, 20].

For stroke prevention in atrial fibrillation, rivaroxaban prescribing information recommends a dose reduction to 15 mg (from 20 mg) when the CrCL falls between 15 and 50 mL/min [3]. This recommendation is made based on pharmacokinetic modeling because patients with CrCL less than 30 mL/min were excluded from the phase III clinical trial that led to the approval of rivaroxaban. Rivaroxaban is contraindicated when CrCL is less than 15 and 30 mL/min for use in atrial fibrillation and prevention of venous thromboembolism after major orthopedic surgery, respectively [3]. Apixaban prescribing information for the EU recommends avoiding apixaban in patients with CrCL <15 mL/min, and urges caution with CrCL is <30 mL/min [20]. Many patients who may benefit from rivaroxaban and apixaban are likely to have renal function near these cut-off points, a fact that emphasizes the importance of ongoing renal function monitoring during this use of these drugs. Renal function influences both the timing of warfarin initiation when transitioning patients from rivaroxaban or apixaban to warfarin as well as the day of discontinuation of rivaroxaban or apixiban prior to invasive procedures [3, 20].

Despite a relatively short half-life (5 to 9 h in healthy volunteers), rivaroxaban is dosed once daily [3]. Clinical trials evaluating apixaban have used twice-daily dosing despite a half-life of 12 h [42]. Quick offset of anticoagulant effect can be viewed as both an advantage (in the setting of interrupting anticoagulation for surgery or invasive procedures) and disadvantage (possible increased risk of therapeutic failure associated with a missed dose) compared to warfarin [3].

Direct Thrombin Inhibitors

Parenteral direct thrombin inhibitors lepirudin, bivalirudin, and argatroban have relatively short half-lives [23–25]. As lepirudin is almost exclusively eliminated via the kidneys, renal function should be estimated prior to administration. In case of renal impairment (CrCL <60 mL/min or serum creatinine >1.5 mg/dL), the initial dose and infusion rate must be reduced. The manufacturer of lepirudin announced in May 2012 that they will no longer produce this medication. Careful titration of anticoagulant effect using the aPTT is recommended [24]. The bivalirudin loading dose does not need to be modified for patients with renal insufficiency, but subsequent infusion rates should be reduced based on the degree of renal dysfunction [25]. Argatroban is cleared primary via hepatic metabolism and biliary secretion and should be considered when parenteral anticoagulation is needed and severe renal insufficiency and heparin intolerance or heparin-induced thrombocytopenia is present. Dose reduction of argatroban is required in the setting of severe liver disease [23].

Dabigatran is also primarily eliminated by the kidneys and assessing renal function before and during therapy is very important. Dose reduction is recommended when CrCL is less than 30 mL/min [22]. Like rivaroxaban, dabigatran has yet to be studied in patients with CrCL less than 30 mL/min. The 75 mg twice daily dose approved by the FDA for patients with CrCL between 15 and 30 mL/min was not evaluated during clinical trials and is derived from pharmacokinetic modeling [22]. The degree of renal function impairment can also influence susceptibility to P-gp-inhibition drug interactions. According to prescribing information, reducing the dose of dabigatran to 75 mg twice daily should be considered when dronedarone or systemic ketoconazole is coadministered in patients with CrCL 30–50 mL/min, and the use of dabigatran in combination with P-gp inhibitors in patients with CrCL 15–30 mL/min should be avoided [22]. As there is no antidote to reverse the anticoagulant effect of dabigatran, removal by dialysis can be an important consideration in the management of life-threatening bleeding caused by dabigatran [22, 23]. While parenteral direct thrombin inbitors are also dialyzable, their short half-lives obviate the need for an antidote or a mechanism for urgent removal.

Dabigatran is dosed twice daily for stroke prevention in atrial fibrillation due to its short half-life [22]. Theoretical advantages and disadvantages (compared to warfarin) related to offset of anticoagulant effect are similar to those previously described for rivaroxaban and apixaban.

Vitamin K Antagonists

Warfarin is metabolized hepatically via CYP enzymes [31]. Warfarin exists as a racemic mixture of two enantiomers, (S) and (R). The more potent S-warfarin is metabolized by CYP 2C9, whereas R-warfarin is metabolized by CYP 1A2 and CYP 3A4. Inactive warfarin metabolites are excreted in both urine and stool. The half-life of warfarin is approximately 40 h with an average duration of anticoagulant activity ranging from 2 to 5 days [31]. The slow offset (and onset) of warfarin's anticoagulant effect complicates interrupting therapy for invasive procedures. Cross coverage with injectable anticoagulants, like UFH or LMWH during the unavoidable period of subtherapeutic anticoagulation (usually several days) associated with stopping and restarting warfarin has been recommended for patients at high risk of thromboembolism [43]. Acenocoumarol and phenprocoumon, vitamin K antagonists used in some jurisdictions, also exist as racemic mixtures. S-acenocoumarol is metabolized quickly by CYP 2C9 (half-life 0.5 h) whereas the more potent R-acenocoumarol has a half-life of 9 h and is metabolized primary by CYP 2C9 and CYP 2C19 [31]. Daily INR response can be variable due to the short half-life of acenocoumarol. S-phenprocoumon is more potent than R-phenprocoumon, but the half-life of both isomers is roughly 5.5 days; both are metabolized by CYP 2C9 [31]. See Table 3.3 for additional details.

Warfarin metabolism is sensitive to concomitantly administered drugs that either induce or inhibit CYP enzymes, especially CYP 2C9 [44]. Drugs known to induce production of CYP450 enzymes or increase their enzymatic activity can reduce the INR and increase the warfarin dose required to maintain therapeutic effect. Drugs that impair or compete for CYP enzymes increase warfarin sensitivity and can precipitate excessive anticoagulation [44]. Common warfarin drug interactions are summarized in Table 3.4.

Because of the importance of CYP 2C9 in the metabolism of warfarin, this enzyme was an intuitive target for investigation into whether genetics might explain some of the inter-patient variability in warfarin dose response. The wild-type 2C9 allele is identified as CYP 2C9*1; two important and relatively common variants have been identified: CYP 2C9*2 and CYP 2C9*3. Individuals who possess one or more variant alleles have increased warfarin sensitivity and possibly increased risk for bleeding [45].

The identification of CYP 2C9 variants explains some but not all of the inter-patient variability in warfarin dose response. Identification of the gene encoding the target enzyme for warfarin, Vitamin K Epoxide Reductase

TABLE 3.4 Selected warfarin pharmacokinetic drug interactions[a]

Increase warfarin sensitivity		Decrease warfarin sensitivity	
Plasma protein displacement	Inhibition or competition for CYP metabolism	CYP inducers	Decrease absorption
	CYP 2C9	CYP 2C9	
– Sulfamethoxazole	– Amiodarone	– Rifampin	– Cholestyramine
– Valproic acid	– Fluconazole	– Carbamazepine	– Colestipol
	– Lovastatin	– Phenobarbital	
	– Tamoxifen	– Aprepitant	
	– Capecitabine		
	– Sitaxsentan		
	– Flurouracil		
	– Noscapine		
	– Voriconazole		
	– Celecoxib		

CYP 1A2	CYP 1A2
– Cimetidine	– Omeprazole
– Ciprofloxacin	– Phenobarbital
– Erythromycin	
– Tacrine	

CYP 3A4	CYP 3A4
– Erythromycin	– Rifampin
– Cimetidine	– Phenytoin
– Fluoxetine	– Phenobarbital
– Ketoconazole	– Carbamazepine
– Posaconazole	
– Voriconazole	
– Metronidazole	
– Ritonavir	
– Indinavir	
– Mibefradil	
– Noscapine	

Adapted from Hansten and Horn's drug interactions and Coumadin product info

CYP cytochrome P-450 enzyme

[a]Not an all inclusive list, additional significant warfarin interactions exist

Complex 1 (VKORC1), has been identified as an additional genetic source of warfarin dose variation. Patients with wild-type VKORC1 (GG) require higher warfarin doses, on average, than patients with one or more variants (e.g. AG or AA). Overall, genetic polymorphisms in CYP 2C9 and VKORC1 explain 35–50 % of warfarin dose variation [46]. See Table 3.5 for a summary of average warfarin doses across genotypes. Genetic alteration in CYP 2C9 and VKORC1 can influence dose response to acenocoumarol and phenprocoumon as well, however phenprocoumon is less susceptible than warfarin due to its long half-life [31]. Prescribing information for warfarin was updated Aug 2007 to encourage, but not require, the use of pharmacogenetic testing to guide warfarin dose initiation [29]. Several warfarin dosing decision support algorithms integrating genetic information have been developed and tested [47]. So far, the availability of genetic information has failed to improve patient outcomes compared to traditional initiation algorithms that adjust the warfarin dose based on frequent INR testing [31, 47]. Ongoing clinical trials will further explore the hypothesis that pharmacogenetic testing might someday reduce adverse outcomes in patients starting therapy with vitamin K antagonists.

Additional factors known to contribute to variability in patient response to treatment with vitamin K antagonists include: age, body mass index, sex, dietary vitamin K intake, alcohol, and adherence as well as comorbid conditions such as heart failure and liver disease. Awareness of these factors, in addition to early INR response and timely INR recheck, are critical to the successful introduction and therapeutic maintenance of warfarin therapy [48].

Vitamin K is an antidote to warfarin therapy [49]. In addition to interrupting warfarin, asymptomatic patients with INR values greater than 5.0 can be managed with or without supplementation with 1–2.5 mg of oral vitamin K [31]. Bleeding patients require vitamin K 10 mg by given by slow intravenous infusion in addition to transfusion of fresh frozen plasma or prothrombin complex concentrates [31].

TABLE 3.5 Maintenance warfarin dose according to CYP 2C9 and VKORC1 genotypes [29]

| VKORC1 | CYP 2C9 | | | | | |
	*1/*1	*1/*2	*1/*3	*2/*2	*2/*3	*3/*3
GG	5–7 mg	5–7 mg	3–4 mg	3–4 mg	3–4 mg	0.5–2 mg
AG	5–7 mg	3–4 mg	3–4 mg	3–4 mg	0.5–2 mg	0.5–2 mg
AA	3–4 mg	3–4 mg	0.5–2 mg	0.5–2 mg	0.5–2 mg	0.5–2 mg

References

1. Wardrop D, Keeling D. The story of the discovery of heparin and warfarin. Br J Haematol. 2008;141:757–63.
2. Haas S. Oral direct thrombin inhibition: an effective and novel approach for venous thromboembolism. Drugs. 2004;64 Suppl 1:7–16.
3. Rivaroxaban prescribing information. 2011. http://www.xarel-tohcp.com/sites/default/files/pdf/xarelto_0.pdf#zoom=100. Accessed on Aug 13, 2012.
4. Monroe DM, Hoffman M. What does it take to make the perfect clot? Arterioscler Thromb Vasc Biol. 2006;26:41–8.
5. Mann KG, Brummel-Ziedins K, Orfeo T, Butenas S. Models of blood coagulation. Blood Cells Mol Dis. 2006;36:108–17.
6. Crawley JT, Zanardelli S, Chion CK, Lane DA. The central role of thrombin in hemostasis. J Thromb Haemost. 2007;5 Suppl 1:95–101.
7. Lussana F, Dentali F, Ageno W, Kamphuisen PW. Venous thrombosis at unusual sites and the role of thrombophilia. Semin Thromb Hemost. 2007;33:582–7.
8. Garcia D, Libby E, Crowther MA. The new oral anticoagulants. Blood. 2010;115:15–20.
9. Piccini JP, Patel MR, Mahaffey KW, Fox KA, Califf RM. Rivaroxaban, an oral direct factor Xa inhibitor. Expert Opin Investig Drugs. 2008;17:925–37.
10. Hirsh J, Bauer KA, Donati MB, et al. Parenteral anticoagulants: American college of chest physicians evidence-based clinical practice guidelines (8th edition). Chest. 2008;133:141S–59.
11. Young E, Cosmi B, Weitz J, Hirsh J. Comparison of the non-specific binding of unfractionated heparin and low molecular weight heparin (enoxaparin) to plasma proteins. Thromb Haemost. 1993;70:625–30.
12. Warkentin TE, Greinacher A, Koster A, Lincoff AM. Treatment and prevention of heparin-induced thrombocytopenia: American college of chest physicians evidence-based clinical practice guidelines (8th edition). Chest. 2008;133:340S–80.
13. Morris TA, Castrejon S, Devendra G, Gamst AC. No difference in risk for thrombocytopenia during treatment of pulmonary embolism and deep venous thrombosis with either low-molecular-weight heparin or unfractionated heparin: a metaanalysis. Chest. 2007;132:1131–9.

14. Casele H, Haney EI, James A, Rosene-Montella K, Carson M. Bone density changes in women who receive thromboprophylaxis in pregnancy. Am J Obstet Gynecol. 2006;195:1109–13.

15. Al-Yaseen E, Wells PS, Anderson J, Martin J, Kovacs MJ. The safety of dosing dalteparin based on actual body weight for the treatment of acute venous thromboembolism in obese patients. J Thromb Haemost. 2005;3:100–2.

16. Clark NP. Low-molecular-weight heparin use in the obese, elderly, and in renal insufficiency. Thromb Res. 2008;123 Suppl 1:S58–61.

17. Bauer KA, Hawkins DW, Peters PC, et al. Fondaparinux, a synthetic pentasaccharide: the first in a new class of antithrombotic agents - the selective factor Xa inhibitors. Cardiovasc Drug Rev. 2002;20:37–52.

18. Warkentin TE, Pai M, Sheppard JI, et al. Fondaparinux treatment of acute heparin-induced thrombocytopenia confirmed by the serotonin-release assay: a 30-month, 16-patient case series. J Thromb Haemost. 2011;9:2389–96.

19. Glaeser H. Importance of P-glycoprotein for drug-drug interactions. Handb Exp Pharmacol. 2011;201:285–97.

20. Apixaban prescribing information. 2011. http://www.eliquis.eu/PDF/ELIQUIS®SmPC.pdf. Accessed on Aug 13, 2012.

21. Raghavan N, Frost CE, Yu Z, et al. Apixaban metabolism and pharmacokinetics after oral administration to humans. Drug Metab Dispos. 2009;37:74–81.

22. Dabigatran prescribing information. 2011. http://bidocs.boehringer-ingelheim.com/BIWebAccess/ViewServlet.ser?docBase=renetnt&folderPath=/Prescribing%20Information/PIs/Pradaxa/Pradaxa.pdf. Accessed on Aug 13, 2012.

23. Agratroban prescribing information. 2011. http://us.gsk.com/products/assets/us_argatroban.pdf. Accessed on Aug 13, 2012.

24. Lepirudin prescribing information. 2011. http://www.accessdata.fda.gov/drugsatfda_docs/label/2006/020807s011lbl.pdf. Accessed on Aug 13, 2012.

25. Bivalirudin prescribing information. 2011. http://www.angiomax.com/Downloads/Angiomax_PI_2010_PN1601-12.pdf. Accessed on Aug 13, 2012.

26. Deitcher SR, Ngengwe R, Kaplan R, et al. Subcutaneous lepirudin for heparin-induced thrombocytopenia and when other anticoagulants fail: illustrative cases. Clin Adv Hematol Oncol. 2004;2: 382–4.

27. Inman KR, Gerlach AT. Use of subcutaneous lepirudin in an obese surgical intensive care unit patient with heparin resistance. Ann Pharmacother. 2009;43:1714–8.
28. Salmela B, Nordin A, Vuoristo M, et al. Budd-Chiari syndrome in a young female with factor V Leiden mutation: successful treatment with lepirudin, a direct thrombin inhibitor. Thromb Res. 2008;121:769–72.
29. Warfarin prescribing information. 2011. http://packageinserts.bms.com/pi/pi_coumadin.pdf. Accessed on Aug 13, 2012.
30. Hansten PD, Horn JR. Drug interactions analysis and management. St. Louis: Wolters Kluwer Health; 2012.
31. Ansell J, Hirsh J, Hylek E, et al. Pharmacology and management of the vitamin K antagonists: American college of chest physicians evidence-based clinical practice guidelines (8th edition). Chest. 2008;133:160S–98.
32. Ahmed A, Stephens JC, Kaus CA, Fay WP. Impact of preemptive warfarin dose reduction on anticoagulation after initiation of trimethoprim-sulfamethoxazole or levofloxacin. J Thromb Thrombolysis. 2008;26:44–8.
33. Clark SL, Porter TF, West FG. Coumarin derivatives and breast-feeding. Obstet Gynecol. 2000;95:938–40.
34. Kaminsky LS, Zhang ZY. Human P450 metabolism of warfarin. Pharmacol Ther. 1997;73:67–74.
35. Lim W, Dentali F, Eikelboom JW, Crowther MA. Meta-analysis: low-molecular-weight heparin and bleeding in patients with severe renal insufficiency. Ann Intern Med. 2006;144:673–84.
36. Spinler SA, Inverso SM, Cohen M, et al. Safety and efficacy of unfractionated heparin versus enoxaparin in patients who are obese and patients with severe renal impairment: analysis from the ESSENCE and TIMI 11B studies. Am Heart J. 2003;146:33–41.
37. Nagge J, Crowther M, Hirsh J. Is impaired renal function a contraindication to the use of low-molecular-weight heparin? Arch Intern Med. 2002;162:2605–9.
38. Enoxaparin prescribing information. 2011. http://products.sanofi.us/lovenox/lovenox.html. Accessed on Aug 13, 2012.
39. Dalteparin prescribing information. 2011. http://www.pfizer.com/files/products/uspi_fragmin.pdf. Accessed on Aug 13, 2012.
40. Kitchen S, Iampietro R, Woolley AM, Preston FE. Anti Xa monitoring during treatment with low molecular weight heparin or danaparoid: inter-assay variability. Thromb Haemost. 1999;82:1289–93.

41. Fondaparinux prescribing information. 2011. http://us.gsk.com/products/assets/us_arixtra.pdf. Accessed on Aug 13, 2012.
42. Patel MR, Mahaffey KW, Garg J, et al. Rivaroxaban versus warfarin in nonvalvular atrial fibrillation. N Engl J Med. 2011;365:883–91.
43. Douketis JD, Berger PB, Dunn AS, et al. The perioperative management of antithrombotic therapy: American college of chest physicians evidence-based clinical practice guidelines (8th edition). Chest. 2008;133:299S–339.
44. Holbrook AM, Pereira JA, Labiris R, et al. Systematic overview of warfarin and its drug and food interactions. Arch Intern Med. 2005;165:1095–106.
45. Higashi MK, Veenstra DL, Kondo LM, et al. Association between CYP2C9 genetic variants and anticoagulation-related outcomes during warfarin therapy. JAMA. 2002;287:1690–8.
46. Gage BF, Eby C, Johnson JA, et al. Use of pharmacogenetic and clinical factors to predict the therapeutic dose of warfarin. Clin Pharmacol Ther. 2008;84:326–31.
47. Kangelaris KN, Bent S, Nussbaum RL, Garcia DA, Tice JA. Genetic testing before anticoagulation? A systematic review of pharmacogenetic dosing of warfarin. J Gen Intern Med. 2009;24:656–64.
48. Garcia DA. Warfarin and pharmacogenomic testing: the case for restraint. Clin Pharmacol Ther. 2008;84:303–5.
49. Crowther MA, Ageno W, Garcia D, et al. Oral vitamin K versus placebo to correct excessive anticoagulation in patients receiving warfarin: a randomized trial. Ann Intern Med. 2009;150:293–300.
50. Unfractionated heparin prescribing information. 2011. http://www.hospira.com/Files/heparin_sodium_injection.pdf. Accessed on Aug 13, 2012.

Chapter 4
Antithrombotic Treatment of Cardiovascular Disease

Jonathan Watt, Jesse Dawson, and Adrian J.B. Brady

Primary Prevention of Cardiovascular Disease

The primary prevention of cardiovascular disease depends on the treatment of modifiable risk factors together with healthy diet and lifestyle. Principally this involves plenty of exercise, a low cholesterol diet, and appropriate treatment of high blood pressure and dyslipidaemia, together with the avoidance of diabetes.

J. Watt, M.D., MRCP (✉)
West of Scotland Regional Heart & Lung Centre,
Golden Jubilee National Hospital,
Agamemnon Street, G81 4DY Glasgow, UK
e-mail: j.watt@nhs.net

J. Dawson, M.D., B.Sc. (Hons), MBChB (Hons), FRCP
Institute of Cardiovascular and Medical Sciences, College of Medicine,
Veterinary & Life Sciences, University of Glasgow, Western Infirmary,
Glasgow, UK
e-mail: jesse.dawson@glasgow.ac.uk

A.J.B. Brady, M.D., FRCP, FESC, FAHA
Department of Medical Cardiology, University of Glasgow,
84 Castle Street, G4 0SF Glasgow, UK
e-mail: a.j.brady@clinmed.gla.ac.uk

A. Ferro, D.A. Garcia (eds.), *Antiplatelet and Anticoagulation*   143
Therapy, Current Cardiovascular Therapy,
DOI 10.1007/978-1-4471-4297-3_4,
© Springer-Verlag London 2013

Benefits and Risks of Aspirin Therapy in Primary Prevention

Antiplatelet therapy has for many years been assumed to be an important part of primary prevention. New data, however, has cast considerable doubt on this widely held belief [1]. Aspirin reduces the risk of myocardial infarction (MI) by about 30%, but increases the risk of haemorrhagic stroke by 40%, and of major gastrointestinal bleeding by 70%. All cause mortality is not improved by aspirin therapy.

Therefore, for 1,000 patients with a 10% risk of cardiovascular (CV) events over 10 years, aspirin would prevent 12–14 MIs but would cause up to four haemorrhagic strokes, and ≤8 major GI bleeds. Therefore, any protection of aspirin is offset by the risks of bleeding. Thus the benefit is defined by the overall risk of cardiovascular events for the individual.

The balance where benefit of aspirin outweighs the risks and bleeding is around 15% CV risk in 10 years. This is roughly similar to the 20% 10 year risk band used by many cardiovascular guidelines as the threshold for treatment of asymptomatic individuals without established CV disease [2]. So for those with a calculated 10 year risk >20%, aspirin 75 mg per day should be considered, after due consideration of the bleeding risks. For patients allergic to aspirin, clopidogrel 75 mg (judged in the absence of a major primary prevention trial) is an alternative.

Surprisingly, for patients with diabetes there is remarkably little evidence of any benefit of aspirin in primary prevention. This is currently being addressed in a large prospective clinical trial, the ASCEND trial (http://www.ctsu.ox.ac.uk/ascend/). This study will report in 2018. So at the moment the pragmatic decision is that for individuals in good health but with diabetes, the 10 year CV risk should be calculated and if >20%, aspirin therapy should be initiated.

Of course, aspirin does offer other benefits, for example a reduction in bowel cancer risk among patients with polyposis coli [3]. For such individuals aspirin is probably a valuable drug, despite the small excess bleeding risk.

Patients with Hypertension

Patients with uncontrolled high blood pressure have a high risk of cerebral haemorrhage and should not receive antiplatelet therapy until the BP is reduced to <150/90 mmHg [2].

Acute Coronary Syndromes

The Dynamic Process of Acute Coronary Occlusion

The pathophysiology of acute coronary syndromes (ACS) is now widely understood to be related to the rupture or erosion of a coronary artery atherosclerotic plaque in the vast majority of cases. Coronary plaque instability leads to superimposed thrombus formation which causes coronary artery obstruction and downstream myocardial ischaemia or infarction. ACS is sub-classified based on the presence or absence of ST segment elevation on the patient's electrocardiogram. This distinction is clinically important because in most cases ST elevation represents complete thrombotic occlusion of a coronary artery, leading to ST elevation myocardial infarction (STEMI), which requires emergency reperfusion strategies without delay.

Non-ST elevation ACS is typically present in patients with incomplete coronary artery occlusion, leading to a diagnosis of unstable angina or non-ST elevation myocardial infarction (NSTEMI), depending on whether myocardial necrosis occurs. Given that ACS is almost always caused by some degree of occlusive coronary thrombosis, antiplatelet and anticoagulant agents constitute the mainstay of drug therapy. For those patients who undergo invasive treatments, notably percutaneous coronary intervention (PCI), intensive antithrombotic therapy is crucial. A wide range of traditional and novel drugs is now available, supported by evidence from major clinical trials. The specific platelet or coagulation targets for these antithrombotic drugs are shown in Fig. 4.1.

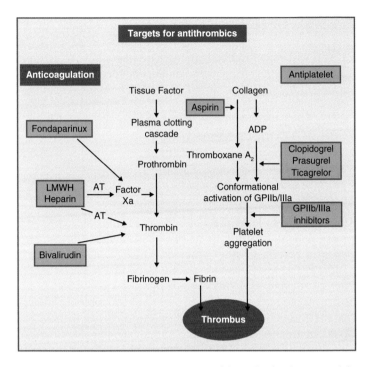

FIGURE 4.1 The primary target for antithrombotic drugs used in ACS (With kind permission of Wright RS, Mayo Clinic)

Although many of these treatments provide benefit throughout the evolution of ACS, it is worth considering their specific use during the immediate, invasive and 12 month convalescence periods post ACS.

Immediate Treatment of Acute Coronary Syndromes

Aspirin

Aspirin is strongly recommended for all patients presenting with non-ST elevation ACS, based on evidence from the Antithrombotic Trialists Collaboration, which demonstrated a major reduction in the rate of vascular events [1]. ISIS-2 provided definitive data for early aspirin use in STEMI patients, with reductions in vascular death, stroke and MI during the first month of treatment [4]. For the treatment of ACS, a loading dose of 300 mg plain aspirin (not enteric coated) should be chewed to accelerate the onset of action. Aspirin should be administered by paramedics or the first health care provider as soon as ACS is suspected, unless there are contraindications. It has now been shown that daily low dose aspirin (75–100 mg) for longer term treatment is as effective as higher doses with a lower incidence of minor bleeding and gastrointestinal intolerance [5,6]. Despite the development of newer, potent antiplatelet medications, aspirin remains a cornerstone of ACS treatment due to its low cost, reliable efficacy and acceptable tolerability.

Clopidogrel

The administration of oral antiplatelet therapy in addition to aspirin (known as dual antiplatelet therapy, DAPT) is now standard in the management of ACS. The first antiplatelet agent to gain attention in this respect was the thienopyridine, clopidogrel. The CURE study found that adding clopidogrel to aspirin in patients with non-ST elevation ACS significantly reduced refractory ischaemia and MI [7], with benefits emerging within 24 h of treatment, at the expense of a small but significant increase in major bleeding [8]. In patients presenting with STEMI, early clopidogrel treatment improved infarct-related artery patency in the CLARITY study [9]. If STEMI is managed non-invasively, oral clopidogrel should also be given, based on data from the COMMIT trial which demonstrated a significant reduction in overall mortality and major vascular events following intravenous fibrinolysis after only 2 weeks of treatment [10]. As clopidogrel requires several hours to exert its full effect, it should be given at the first opportunity and many ambulance personnel now routinely administer a loading dose of clopidogrel to STEMI patients.

Prasugrel

Prasugrel is a more potent thienopyridine with a faster onset of action. Like clopidogrel, prasugrel should be administered using an oral loading dose following by maintenance therapy. The TRITON-TIMI 38 clinical trial randomised patients with moderate to high risk ACS requiring PCI, to prasugrel or clopidogrel [11]. A landmark analysis of TRITON-TIMI 38 demonstrated that prasugrel reduced MI and urgent target revascularisation within 3 days of treatment, with a small but non-significant increase in major bleeding during this time period [12]. Owing to its potent and rapid antiplatelet effects in patients undergoing PCI [13], prasugrel is now given in some hospitals in place of clopidogrel for the treatment of STEMI prior to emergency angiography.

Ticagrelor

Ticagrelor is an oral antiplatelet drug which acts in a similar fashion to the thienopyridines but is differentiated by its reversible action on platelet ADP receptors. It has similar potency and rapidity of onset compared to prasugrel but a shorter half-life, therefore needs to be administered twice daily. The PLATO study [14] assessed the benefit of ticagrelor over clopidogrel and demonstrated a decrease in vascular death, MI or stroke within 30 days. The safety of ticagrelor was acceptable amongst trial participants, with a very small increase in fatal intracranial bleeding but no significant increase in major bleeding overall. Within the first week of therapy, asymptomatic ventricular pauses were increased but these resolved after 1 month and did not require any specific treatment. Ticagrelor is given as a loading dose of 180 mg followed by 90 mg twice daily. It is likely that ticagrelor will compete with prasugrel to replace clopidogrel in ACS due to improved ischaemic efficacy, but this should be considered in relation to increased prescribing costs and the potential risk of bleeding in individual patients.

Heparins

Both unfractionated and low molecular weight heparin (LMWH) have been shown to offer major benefits in patients with non-ST elevation ACS by halving the risk of death or MI versus placebo [15]. Unfractionated heparin is now rarely used unless serious bleeding is a concern, when it can be rapidly reversed if needed. Compared with unfractionated heparin, enoxaparin provides only small incremental benefits in ACS [16], but it is preferred due to its ease of administration. Predictably, the most common serious adverse effect of enoxaparin is bleeding, which is significantly increased in renal failure due to the risk of accumulation and the dose should be halved in these cases.

Fondaparinux

Fondaparinux is an indirect factor Xa inhibitor which may be used during ACS as an alternative to heparin or LMWH. In the OASIS-5 study, a fixed 2.5 mg subcutaneous dose in patients with non-ST elevation ACS provided similar efficacy to enoxaparin, with a lower incidence of serious bleeding (Fig. 4.2) [17]. This improved safety profile, most notable in patients at increased risk of bleeding due to advanced age or renal impairment, was probably responsible for decreasing mortality during longer term follow-up. Many centres now routinely administer fondaparinux for the medical treatment of ACS in place of unfractionated heparin or LMWH.

Fibrinolytic Therapy

Prior to the widespread adoption of invasive strategies to manage ACS, intravenous fibrinolysis was commonly used as a primary treatment for STEMI, ideally within 6 h of presentation. Fibrinolysis improves survival in medically managed patients with STEMI [4]. Furthermore, intravenous

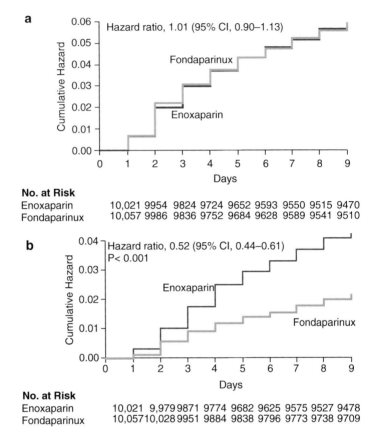

FIGURE 4.2 The OASIS-5 trial in patients with ACS showed that fondaparinux was equivalent to enoxaparin in terms of death, MI or refractory ischemia (panel **a**), but reduced the incidence of serious bleeding after 9 days (panel **b**)

fibrinolysis administered very early in the time course of STEMI (within the first 2 h) may still be the preferred coronary reperfusion strategy for patients who are likely to experience delays prior to accessing invasive treatment [18]. No benefit has ever been demonstrated using fibrinolysis in non-ST elevation ACS.

Specific Issues Related to an Invasive ACS Strategy

An invasive strategy in ACS refers to early coronary angiography and coronary revascularisation in anatomically suitable patients. In the majority of cases, revascularisation is achieved by PCI, whereas a small proportion of patients require coronary artery bypass graft surgery (CABG). Meta-analysis has demonstrated that in patients with non-ST elevation ACS, a routine invasive strategy significantly reduces angina, MI and death compared with a selectively invasive approach [19]. In STEMI patients, PCI reduces MI stroke and death compared to fibrinolysis [20]. Due to the intensely thrombogenic nature of PCI, particularly in the setting of ACS, potent antithrombotic regimens are necessary and merit specific consideration.

Oral Antiplatelet Therapy During PCI

Clopidogrel and aspirin should be given prior to PCI for the treatment of ACS. PCI-CURE showed that pre-treatment of clopidogrel before PCI in non-ST elevation ACS leads to a reduction in cardiovascular death or MI [21]. Similar findings were reported in the PCI-CLARITY study in STEMI patients who underwent PCI after fibrinolysis [22]. Although a 300 mg clopidogrel loading dose was used in early ACS trials, 600 mg provides more rapid and potent antiplatelet effects and is now standard for all patients undergoing emergency coronary angiography, unless fibrinolysis has also been given [23]. A major benefit of intensifying oral antiplatelet treatment prior to PCI for ACS is the prevention of stent thrombosis, which carries a high risk of MI and death (Fig. 4.3). By doubling the dose of clopidogrel for 1 week [6], or switching to a more potent antiplatelet drug such as prasugrel [12] or ticagrelor [24], the risk of stent thrombosis after PCI for ACS is approximately halved. In patients with ACS who require emergency CABG, ticagrelor may offer improved protection

152   J. Watt et al.

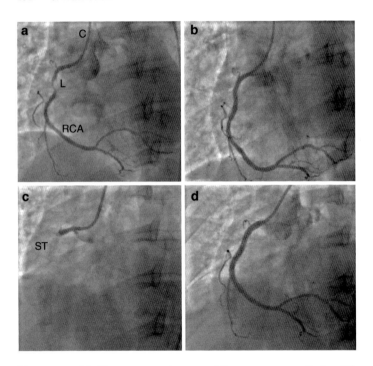

FIGURE 4.3 (**a**) Coronary angiogram with a coronary catheter (C) placed at the ostium of the right coronary artery (RCA) with a stenotic lesion (L). (**b**) Angiographic result following dilation of the lesion and coronary stent implantation. (**c**) Repeat angiogram several days later shows an early stent thrombosis (ST) with occlusive thrombus blocking the stent, which caused a large MI. (**d**) Final angiographic result after the stent thrombosis has been treated using thrombus aspiration and further stenting

against ischaemia and perioperative bleeding due to its reversibility [25].

Glycoprotein IIb/IIIa Receptor Inhibitors

Early trials of intravenous glycoprotein IIb/IIIa receptor inhibitors (GP IIb/IIIa receptor inhibitors) demonstrated clinical efficacy in patients with ACS, however subgroup analysis has shown that the benefits are virtually entirely confined to those patients treated invasively [26]. Contemporary studies have suggested that routine abciximab use during primary PCI for STEMI may be less effective if patients have been adequately preloaded with high dose clopidogrel [27], although prehospital treatment with high dose tirofiban does still appear to benefit these patients [28]. Clinical trials directly comparing GP IIb/IIIa receptor inhibitors suggest that high dose tirofiban has similar efficacy to abciximab [29], whereas no reliable comparative data is available for eptifibitide. Taken together, these data support a role for early treatment using intravenous GP IIb/IIIa receptor inhibitors (ideally high dose tirofiban or abciximab) for high risk patients undergoing PCI for ACS who are at low risk of bleeding. The clinical benefit of GP IIb/IIIa receptor inhibitors in STEMI is likely to be greater if patients are not adequately pretreated with oral DAPT, which is commonly an issue in clinical practice.

Anticoagulants

Parenteral anticoagulants are mandatory during the invasive treatment of ACS. Although unfractionated heparin is still commonly used, there is understandable enthusiasm surrounding the use of more specific and reliable novel anticoagulants. In non-ST elevation ACS, subcutaneous enoxaparin was shown to be equivalent to unfractionated heparin in the SYNERGY trial in terms of ischaemic endpoints, but led to a modest increase in serious bleeding [30]. The OASIS trial program showed that fondaparinux was responsible for a higher rate of catheter thrombosis in patients managed invasively with non-ST elevation ACS [17] and, to an even greater extent, STEMI [31]. For this reason, an intravenous bolus of unfractionated heparin is given to patients treated with fondaparinux who subsequently undergo invasive management for ACS.

Bivalirudin

The direct thrombin inhibitor bivalirudin is a viable alternative to heparin + GP IIb/IIIa receptor inhibitor during the invasive management of ACS, principally because of a lesser bleeding risk [32]. The HORIZONS-AMI study randomised patients with STEMI to bivalirudin or a combination of heparin and GP IIb/IIIa receptor inhibitor and found that bivalirudin reduced mortality, MI and major bleeding (Fig 4.4) [33]. As a result of these favourable data, bivalirudin is now used in many centres during primary PCI in place of more traditional antithombotic regimens.

Post ACS to 12 months

Clopidogrel

The CURE data demonstrated that DAPT using aspirin and clopidogrel following ACS was effective if continued for up to 12 months [7]. The principal benefit of adding clopidogrel for this period was a reduction in MI, with no improvement in mortality and a small increase in serious bleeding. In patients with ACS who have undergone PCI, prolonged treatment with DAPT is essential to protect against late stent thrombosis, which is not sufficiently averted by aspirin alone or anticoagulant drugs.

Prasugrel

The TRITON-TIMI 38 study showed that following 1 year of treatment after PCI for ACS, prasugrel was more effective than clopidogrel in improving ischaemic outcomes, primarily by reducing non-fatal MI (Fig 4.5) [11]. However, this was at the cost of a significant increase in serious bleeding. Fatal cardiovascular events and fatal bleeding were

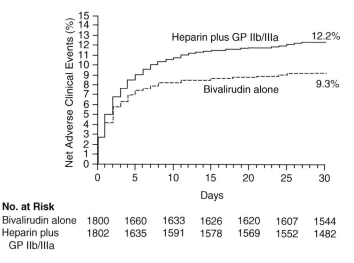

FIGURE 4.4 In the HORIZONS-AMI trial in patients with STEMI, bivalirudin versus heparin and GP IIb/IIIa receptor inhibitor reduced the primary endpoint of net adverse clinical events (defined as major bleeding, death, MI, target-vessel revascularisation for ischaemia, and stroke) (9.2 vs. 12.1%; relative risk, 0.76; 95% confidence interval 0.63–0.92; p=0.005), driven by a significant reduction in major bleeding (4.9 vs. 8.3%; relative risk, 0.60; 95% confidence interval, 0.46–0.77; p<0.001)

counterbalanced in equal measure, hence overall mortality was unchanged. Interestingly, the risk-benefit of prasugrel appeared to specifically favour diabetic patients, who may be at higher ischaemic risk relative to their risk of bleeding. On the other hand, those at increased risk of bleeding, such as the elderly or low body weight, assume an unacceptable risk-benefit profile if prasugrel is used and so it should be avoided in these patients. It may be reasonable consider prasugrel in diabetic patients undergoing PCI for ACS, in patients with stent thrombosis or in the event of clopidogrel intolerance.

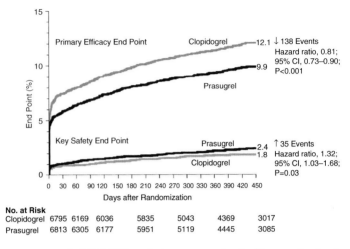

FIGURE 4.5 The TRITON study demonstrated a significant reduction in the primary efficacy endpoint (cardiovascular death, non-fatal MI, non-fatal stroke) using prasugrel versus clopidogrel after PCI for ACS. There was a small increase in the key safety endpoint (major bleeding unrelated to CABG) in the prasugrel group

Ticagrelor

The PLATO study [14] showed that ticagrelor significantly reduced MI and vascular death compared to clopidogrel following 1 year of treatment after ACS (Fig 4.6). Fatal bleeding was similar and so overall mortality was reduced by ticagrelor. Unlike the TRITON-TIMI 38 study testing prasugrel, a fifth of patients in PLATO received a 600 mg loading dose of clopidogrel (reflecting contemporary practice) and this did not negate the benefit of ticagrelor. Breathlessness was reported during follow-up more frequently in patients taking ticagrelor, but this was reversible after drug discontinuation and not associated with a decline in lung function. In the PLATO study, the benefits of ticagrelor were consistent whether or not the patient was invasively or medically managed. There is yet no trial directly comparing ticagrelor versus prasugrel.

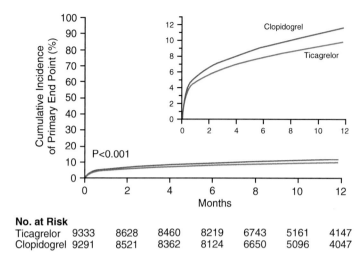

No. at Risk							
Ticagrelor	9333	8628	8460	8219	6743	5161	4147
Clopidogrel	9291	8521	8362	8124	6650	5096	4047

FIGURE 4.6 The PLATO trial confirmed a significant benefit in the primary endpoint (vascular death, myocardial infarction or stroke) using ticagrelor versus clopidogrel after ACS (hazard ratio, 0.84; 95 % confidence interval, 0.77–0.92; $p < 0.001$)

Oral Direct Factor IIa and Xa Inhibitors

These new drugs, likely to gradually replace warfarin in AF and DVT/PE management, have been an attractive prospect in ACS. Dabigatran, rivaroxaban and apixaban have all been tested. Dabigatran [34] and apixaban [35] have not shown any benefit, and both caused an excess of serious bleeding. Rivaroxaban in a low dose has demonstrated a small additional benefit over conventional therapy, but at the expense of more bleeding [36]. None is yet licensed for ACS use. We are reminded that warfarin offered limited benefits in ACS [37].

Suggested Antithrombotic Treatment in ACS

Taking into consideration the most contemporary clinical trial data, a treatment algorithm for ACS can be devised (Fig 4.7). International societies have published similar

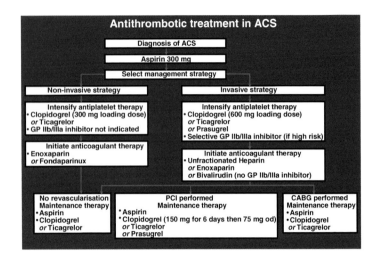

FIGURE 4.7 Suggested antithrombotic treatment in ACS based on management strategy (Modified from Wright et al. [39] ACC/AHA STEMI guidelines)

recommendations [38,39]. Strategies for individual patients will vary, especially depending on the type of ACS, the estimated risk of recurrent ischaemia versus the risk of bleeding, and local financial constraints.

Longer term Secondary Prevention of Cardiovascular Disease

Coronary Heart Disease

The four cornerstones of secondary prevention are: beta-blockers and ACE inhibitors post MI; statins; and anti-platelet therapy. There is also abundant evidence for a large protective benefit of rehabilitation, with a healthy Mediterranean-type diet and a graded exercise programme, and these benefits should not be overlooked [2].

The benefit of antiplatelet therapy is well established. Aspirin reduces all cause mortality, vascular mortality, non-fatal recurrent MI and non-fatal stroke. Patients with established cardiovascular disease should be treated with 75 mg of aspirin daily. Those intolerant of aspirin or who have aspirin allergy should receive clopidogrel 75 mg [2].

Peripheral Arterial Disease

Antiplatelet therapy reduces subsequent ischaemic cardio-vascular events or vascular death by about 25%. Aspirin 75 mg is recommended for all patients with peripheral arterial disease. Clopidogrel 75 mg is at least as effective as aspirin and is a suitable alternative [2].

Treatment of Acute Stroke

For ischaemic stroke, proven effective interventions include stroke unit care, aspirin, and reperfusion therapy with intra-venous thrombolytic therapy. Intra-arterial thrombolysis is of benefit in a small subset of patients with large artery occlusion and ischaemic stroke. For intracerebral haemorrhage, there is no specific licensed or effective treatment beyond stroke unit care.

Antiplatelet and Anticoagulant Drugs

Antiplatelet therapy reduces risk of death if given early after acute ischaemic stroke. This has been confirmed in two large randomised clinical trials and in a systematic review and meta-analysis (n = 43,041). For every 1,000 patients treated acutely with aspirin (160–300 mg) there were 13 fewer deaths [40]. UK guidelines recommend that patients with acute ischaemic stroke are given aspirin 300 mg daily for 2 weeks, followed by an appropriate secondary preventative antiplatelet strategy [41,42]. In patients unable to take aspirin, alternatives eg. clopidogrel may be used. There is no evidence to support the use of early anticoagulation as a treatment for acute ischaemic stroke [43], but this is indicated for the prevention of cardioembolic stroke.

Thrombolysis for Acute Ischaemic Stroke

Use of alteplase, an intravenous tissue plasminogen activator (rt-PA) is beneficial if given within 4.5 h following acute ischaemic stroke in selected patients. The European licence for rt-PA restricts use to within 3 h of symptom onset, although many routinely treat patients up to 4.5 h [44]. Use of rt-PA leads to a reduction in longer term disability, with a number needed to treat of 3 where disability is measured at 90 days [45]. The number needed to treat to avoid death or dependency is ≈ 7. Typically rt-PA use does not lead to immediate improvement in neurological impairment, nor lower mortality rates. A pooled meta-analysis [46] of the major thrombolysis trials (n = 2,775) demonstrated the odds of survival with no disability were 2.8 (95 % CI 1.8–9.5) for treatment within 90 min and 1.6 (95 % CI 1.1–2.2) for treatment between 91 and 180 min with a smaller benefit for patients treated between 181 and 270 min (odds ratio 1.4, 95 % CI 1.1–1.9). The rate of significant intracerebral haemorrhage was 5.9 % in those treated with rt-PA compared to 1.1 % in those treated with placebo, although only a small number of these were of clinical significance. Data from the Safe Implementation of Thrombolysis in Stroke-Monitoring Study (SITS-MOST) [47] show comparable results can be obtained in routine clinical practice (Table 4.1).

Difficulties and Risks of Acute Thrombolysis for Stroke

There are several barriers to use of thrombolytic therapy for acute ischaemic stroke. First, the limited time window for delivery renders many patients ineligible. Second, brain

TABLE 4.1 Summary of outcomes in thrombolysis studies and the SITS register

	Mortality (at 3/12) (%)	Independent (at 3/12) (%)	S-ICH (per SITS-MOST)[a]	S-ICH[b] (%)
Trials	17.3	49	N/A	8.6
SITS-MOST	11.3	54.8	1.7%	7.3
Placebo	18.4	30.2	N/A	1.9

[a]Bleed large enough to cause symptoms and accompanying neurological deterioration
[b]Any bleed with any alteration in neurological status regardless of severity

imaging is mandatory prior to treatment to exclude intracerebral haemorrhage and stroke mimics which takes time and finally, stringent patient selection criteria exist to minimise the risk of iatrogenic intracerebral haemorrhage (Table 4.2). It is crucial to note that while treatment is of benefit out to 4.5 h, the odds of survival with no disability are greatest if rt-PA is administered early and given that the prime benefit of rt-PA is in reducing disability, treatment should not be given to those who are already severely functionally impaired. Patients aged over 80 years were excluded from most of the clinical trials and although they are not covered by the licence, observational data suggests they derive similar benefit [48].

Late Thrombolysis

The benefit (or risk) of treatment beyond 4.5 h is not yet established and it is currently being explored whether use of advanced computed tomography and magnetic resonance imaging sequences can help identify those who will benefit from treatment beyond 4.5 h from onset. Intra-arterial thrombolysis is of benefit [49] in a subset of patients with large artery ischaemic stroke but neither this or mechanical clot retrieval have been adequately studied or compared to intravenous thrombolytic treatment.

TABLE 4.2 Contraindications to the use of rt-PA

General contraindications to any use of rt-PA	Specific contraindications to rt-PA use in ischemic stroke
History of severe bleeding within past 6 months	Evidence of intracranial haemorrhage
Known bleeding diathesis	Onset of symptoms >4.5 h
Oral anticoagulant use (INR>1.4)	Unclear time of onset
History of intracranial haemorrhage	Age <18 or >80 years
Recent (<10 days) CPR	Mild stroke (NIHSS <5)/ rapidly improving
Bacterial endocarditis or pericarditis	Severe stroke (NIHSS >25/ imaging)
Acute Pancreatitis	Seizure at onset of stroke
Recent (<3 months) peptic ulcer disease	Symptoms suggestive of subarachnoid haemorrhage
Neoplasm with bleeding risk	Platelet count < 100,000 per mm³
Recent puncture of non compressible vessel	Heparin within last 48 h with raised PTT
Major surgery or trauma (<3 months)	Prior stroke within last 3 months
Severe liver disease	Prior stroke and concomitant diabetes
Recent obstetric delivery	Systolic BP > 185 or diastolic > 110 mmHg

Prevention of Stroke

Primary Prevention of Stroke

Current preventative strategies include antiplatelet therapy and lipid-lowering therapy to prevent ischaemic stroke, anti-coagulant therapy to prevent cardioembolic stroke, and blood pressure reduction to prevent all stroke types. All stroke survivors should undergo screening for (and treatment of) prevalent diabetes mellitus, smoking cessation therapy, and lifestyle modification. The antithrombotic drugs used to prevent stroke are described below and the main practice changing clinical trials are summarised in Table 4.3.

Antithrombotic Drugs for Secondary Prevention of Non-Cardioembolic Stroke

Antiplatelet Monotherapy

Aspirin prevents up to a fifth of recurrent strokes [1] and most studies suggest an approximate relative risk reduction (RRR) of 15% in comparison with placebo [50] for both recurrent stroke and composite vascular endpoints. For example, in the UK-TIA study [50], 2,435 subjects were enrolled and aspirin treatment (either 300 mg or 1,200 mg per day) led to a 15% relative risk reduction (RRR) in a composite endpoint of vascular death, nonfatal MI and nonfatal stroke. The CAPRIE trial [51] compared clopidogrel monotherapy to aspirin in 19,185 patients with symptomatic cardiovascular disease (recent ischaemic stroke, MI or symptomatic peripheral vascular disease (PVD)). Overall, clopidogrel use gave a small but statistically significant reduction in the occurrence of ischaemic stroke, MI or vascular death (5.32% with clopidogrel compared to 5.83% with aspirin, p=0.043). However, this small 8.7% (95% CI 3–16.5%) RRR was driven by an effect in those with PVD (RRR 23.8%, p=0.0028) and no difference was seen in those with previous stroke and with regard to subsequent stroke risk. Dipyridamole monotherapy provides similar efficacy to aspirin with regard to recurrent stroke prevention, but has no effect on subsequent risk of MI [52].

Dual Antiplatelet Therapy

Aspirin and dipyridamole in combination is superior to placebo and aspirin with regard to recurrent stroke risk [53,54] but benefit on other vascular endpoints is less clear. The recent ESPRIT trial [54] involved 2,763 patients with recent stroke or

TABLE 4.3 Summary of the main anti-platelet trials shaping practice after ischaemic stroke

Trial name n	Population	Comparison	Primary endpoint	Primary efficacy analysis
ATC, n=10,000	Previous stroke/ TIA	Antiplatelet vs. placebo	Vascular event	Reduction in odds of event with anti-platelet 22%, p<0.0001
CAPRIE, n=19 185	Atherosclerotic vascular disease	Clopidogrel vs. aspirin	Ischaemic stroke, MI, vascular death	RRR following clopidogrel 8.7%, 95% CI 0.3–16.5
ESPRIT, n=2,763	Previous TIA or minor stroke taking aspirin	Aspirin and dipyridamole vs. aspirin	Vascular death, stroke, MI, major bleeding complication	HR following aspirin and dipyridamole 0.8, 95% CI 0.68–0.98
CHARISMA, n=15,603	Vascular disease or multiple risk factors	Clopidogrel and aspirin vs. aspirin	Vascular death, MI or stroke.	RRR following clopidogrel and aspirin 0.93, 95% CI 0.83–1.05
MATCH, n=7,599	Recent stroke or TIA	Clopidogrel and aspirin vs. clopidogrel	Vascular death, stroke, MI, or rehospitalisation for an ischaemic event	RRR following clopidogrel and aspirin 6.4%, 95% CI −4.6–16.3
PRoFESS, n=20 332	Previous ischaemic stroke or TIA	Aspirin and dipyridamole vs. clopidogrel	Recurrent stroke	HR following aspirin and dipyridamole 0.99, 95% CI 0.92–1.07

ATC Antiplatelet Trialists Collaboration, *TIA* transient ischaemic attack, *MI* myocardial infarction, *HR* hazard ratio, *RRR* relative risk reduction

TIA and revealed, during a mean follow-up of 3.5 years, that the combination of aspirin and slow-release dipyridamole afford a 20% relative risk reduction (HR 0.8, 95% CI 0.66–0.98, ARR 1% per year) in the rate of vascular death or non-fatal stroke or MI compared to aspirin alone. There was no increase in bleeding complications. The results of ESPRIT confirmed those of the previous ESPS 2 study [53].

The recent PRoFESS study compared aspirin (and modified-release dipyridamole) with clopidogrel and included 20,332 patients with recent stroke [55]. There was no difference between the treatment groups in primary endpoint of recurrent stroke (9% following aspirin and dipyridamole vs. 8.8% following clopidogrel, HR 1.01, 95% CI 0.92–1.11).

The MATCH [56] and CHARISMA trials [57] revealed no extra benefit of aspirin and clopidogrel in combination compared to either agent as monotherapy in those with established vascular disease, including after stroke. However, the combination of aspirin and clopidogrel may be of benefit in certain high risk groups including those with very recent stroke and atrial fibrillation who are unsuitable for anti-coagulation.

Anticoagulant Drugs

For patients in sinus rhythm there is no benefit above that of aspirin therapy from the use of warfarin in those with ischaemic stroke and no evidence of cardioembolic stroke. No other oral anticoagulant has been studied in this setting. The remarkable progress with the new oral antioagulants for patients with atrial fibrillation is discussed in the next chapter.

Antithrombotic Drugs for Cardioembolic Stroke

Atrial Fibrillation

Presence of atrial fibrillation increases risk of both first stroke and recurrent stroke. Scoring algorithms such as the CHADS2 score are now commonly employed to help identify those with atrial fibrillation most likely to benefit from anticoagulant treatment. However, CHADS2 has the disadvantage of underestimating stroke risk in younger patients and the newer CHA2DS2-VASc is now the much preferred risk algorithm.

The most widely used and studied anticoagulant is warfarin, which inhibits synthesis of vitamin K-dependent clotting factors. It is hugely effective. Meta-analysis data show a reduction in stroke rate from 4.5 % per annum to 1.4 % following warfarin treatment [58] with a target INR of range of two to three. It is similarly effective in the secondary preventative setting [59].

Crucially, as well as being inferior in terms of stroke prevention, safety and risk of haemorrhage, aspirin conveys a similar risk of major bleeding rate (≈ 1 % compared to 1.3 % per annum with warfarin).

Dual antiplatelet therapy with aspirin and clopidogrel has been compared to warfarin and offers inferior stroke protection at the cost of a similar burden of bleeding complications but this may be superior to aspirin in those who cannot take warfarin [60].

There are a number of newer oral anticoagulant drugs available which potentially offer considerable advantages over use of warfarin and these are discussed in the following chapter.

Transient Ischaemic Attack (TIA)

The approach to secondary prevention after TIA is the same as for following ischaemic stroke. Patients with TIA were included in many of the aforementioned clinical trials. Given the common pathogensis of TIA and ischaemic stroke, there is little reason therefore to suspect that the evidence base cannot be extrapolated, The most compelling specific evidence that the above treatments are efficacious in TIA comes from the pivotal EXPRESS study, In this trial, early initiation of standard therapy with antiplatelets, blood pressure lowering drugs, statins and

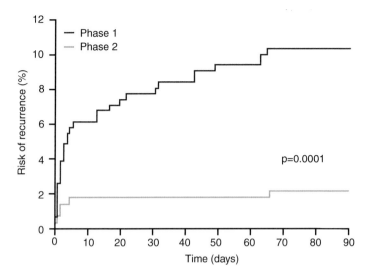

FIGURE 4.8 Risk of recurrent stroke after first seeking medical attention in all patients with TIA or stroke who were referred to the study clinic. Phase two refers to the period of rapid investigation and treatment of TIA compared to phase 1 (standard care)

anticoagulation and carotid surgery where indicated led to an 80% RRR in risk of stroke at 90 days (Fig 4.8) [61].

References

1. Antithrombotic Trialists' Collaboration. Aspirin in the primary and secondary prevention of vascular disease: collaborative meta-analysis of individual participant data from randomised trials. Lancet. 2009;373:1849–60.
2. Grant J, Brady AJB Brindle P, et al. SIGN 97 – risk estimation and the prevention of cardiovascular disease. Edinburgh: Scottish Intercollegiate Guidelines Network; 2007.
3. Burn J, Bishop DT, Chapman PD, et al. A randomized Placebo-controlled prevention trial of aspirin and/or resistant starch in young people with familial adenomatous polyposis. Cancer Prev Res. 2011;4:655–65.

4. ISIS-2 (Second International Study of Infarct Survival) Collaborative Group. Randomised trial of intravenous streptokinase, oral aspirin, both, or neither among 17,187 cases of suspected acute myocardial infarction: ISIS-2. Lancet. 1988;2:349–60.

5. Antithrombotic Trialists' Collaboration. Collaborative meta-analysis of randomised trials of antiplatelet therapy for prevention of death, myocardial infarction, and stroke in high risk patients. BMJ. 2002;324:71–86.

6. Mehta SR, Tanguay JF, Eikelboom JW, et al. Double-dose versus standard-dose clopidogrel and high-dose versus low-dose aspirin in individuals undergoing percutaneous coronary intervention for acute coronary syndromes (CURRENT-OASIS 7): a randomised factorial trial. Lancet. 2010;376:1233–43.

7. Yusuf S, et al. Effects of clopidogrel in addition to aspirin in patients with acute coronary syndromes without ST-segment elevation. N Engl J Med. 2001;345:494–502.

8. Yusuf S, Mehta SR, Zhao F, et al. Early and late effects of clopidogrel in patients with acute coronary syndromes. Circulation. 2003;107:966–72.

9. Sabatine MS, Cannon CP, Gibson CM, et al. Addition of clopidogrel to aspirin and fibrinolytic therapy for myocardial infarction with ST-segment elevation. N Engl J Med. 2005;352:1179–89.

10. Chen ZM, Jiang LX, Chen YP, et al. Addition of clopidogrel to aspirin in 45,852 patients with acute myocardial infarction: randomised placebo-controlled trial. Lancet. 2005;366:1607–21.

11. Wiviott SD, Braunwald E, McCabe CH, et al. Prasugrel versus clopidogrel in patients with acute coronary syndromes. N Engl J Med. 2007;357:2001–15.

12. Antman EM, Wiviott SD, Murphy SA, et al. Early and late benefits of prasugrel in patients with acute coronary syndromes undergoing percutaneous coronary intervention: a TRITON-TIMI 38 (TRial to assess improvement in therapeutic outcomes by optimizing platelet InhibitioN with prasugrel-thrombolysis in myocardial infarction) analysis. J Am Coll Cardiol. 2008;51:2028–33.

13. Wiviott SD, Trenk D, Frelinger AL, et al. Prasugrel compared with high loading- and maintenance-dose clopidogrel in patients with planned percutaneous coronary intervention. Circulation. 2007;116:2923–32.

14. Wallentin L, Becker RC, Budaj A, et al. Ticagrelor versus clopidogrel in patients with acute coronary syndromes. N Engl J Med. 2009;361:1045–57.

15. Eikelboom JW, Anand SS, Malmberg K, Weitz JI, Ginsberg JS, Yusuf S. Unfractionated heparin and low-molecular-weight heparin in acute coronary syndrome without ST elevation: a meta-analysis. Lancet. 2000;355:1936–42.
16. Murphy SA, Gibson CM, Morrow DA, et al. Efficacy and safety of the low-molecular weight heparin enoxaparin compared with unfractionated heparin across the acute coronary syndrome spectrum: a meta-analysis. Eur Heart J. 2007;28:2077–86.
17. Yusuf S, et al. Comparison of fondaparinux and enoxaparin in acute coronary syndromes. N Engl J Med. 2006;354:1464–76.
18. Bonnefoy E, Steg PG, Boutitie F, et al. Comparison of primary angioplasty and pre-hospital fibrinolysis in acute myocardial infarction (CAPTIM) trial: a 5-year follow-up. Eur Heart J. 2009;30: 1598–606.
19. Bavry AA, Kumbhani DJ, Rassi AN, Bhatt DL, Askari AT. Benefit of early invasive therapy in acute coronary syndromes: a meta-analysis of contemporary randomized clinical trials. J Am Coll Cardiol. 2006;48:1319–25.
20. Keeley EC, Boura JA, Grines CL. Primary angioplasty versus intravenous thrombolytic therapy for acute myocardial infarction: a quantitative review of 23 randomised trials. Lancet. 2003;361(9351):13–20.
21. Mehta SR, Yusuf S, Peters RJ, et al. Effects of pretreatment with clopidogrel and aspirin followed by long-term therapy in patients undergoing percutaneous coronary intervention: the PCI-CURE study [abstr]. Lancet. 2001;358:527–33.
22. Sabatine MS, Cannon CP, Gibson CM, et al. Effect of clopidogrel pretreatment before percutaneous coronary intervention in patients with ST-elevation myocardial infarction treated with fibrinolytics. JAMA. 2005;294:1224–32.
23. Patti G, Barczi G, Orlic D, et al. Outcome comparison of 600- and 300-mg loading doses of clopidogrel in patients undergoing primary percutaneous coronary intervention for ST-segment elevation myocardial infarction: results from the ARMYDA-6 MI (antiplatelet therapy for reduction of MYocardial damage during angioplasty-myocardial infarction) randomized study. J Am Coll Cardiol. 2011; 58:1592–9.
24. Cannon CP, Harrington RA, James S, et al. Comparison of ticagrelor with clopidogrel in patients with a planned invasive strategy for acute coronary syndromes (PLATO): a randomised double-blind study [abstr]. Lancet. 2010;375:283–93.

25. Held C, Asenblad N, Bassand JP, et al. Ticagrelor versus clopi-
    dogrel in patients with acute coronary syndromes undergoing
    coronary artery bypass surgery: results from the PLATO (platelet
    inhibition and patient outcomes) trial. J Am Coll Cardiol. 2011;
    57:672–84.
26. Roffi M, Chew DP, Mukherjee D, et al. Platelet glycoprotein IIb/
    IIIa inhibition in acute coronary syndromes. Gradient of benefit
    related to the revascularization strategy. Eur Heart J. 2002;23:
    1441–8.
27. Mehilli J, Kastrati A, Schulz S, et al. Abciximab in patients with
    acute ST-segment elevation myocardial infarction undergoing
    primary percutaneous coronary intervention after clopidogrel
    loading. Circulation. 2009;119:1933–40.
28. Van't Hof AW, ten Berg J, Heestermans T, et al. Prehospital ini-
    tiation of tirofiban in patients with ST-elevation myocardial
    infarction undergoing primary angioplasty (On-TIME 2): a mul-
    ticentre, double-blind, randomised controlled trial. Lancet.
    2008;372:537–46.
29. Valgimigli M, Campo G, Percoco G, et al. Comparison of angio-
    plasty with infusion of tirofiban or abciximab and with implanta-
    tion of sirolimus-eluting or uncoated stents for acute myocardial
    infarction. JAMA. 2008;299:1788–99.
30. Synergy T. I. enoxaparin vs unfractionated heparin in high-risk
    patients with non ST-segment elevation acute coronary syn-
    dromes managed with an intended early invasive strategy.
    JAMA. 2004;292:45–54.
31. Yusuf S, Mehta SR, Chrolavicius S, et al. Effects of fondaparinux
    on mortality and reinfarction in patients with acute ST-segment
    elevation myocardial infarction: the OASIS-6 randomized trial.
    JAMA. 2006;295:1519–30.
32. Stone GW, McLaurin BT, Cox DA, et al. Bivalirudin for patients
    with acute coronary syndromes. N Engl J Med. 2006;355:2203–16.
33. Stone GW, Witzenbichler B, Guagliumi G, et al. Bivalirudin dur-
    ing primary PCI in acute myocardial infarction. N Engl J Med.
    2008;358:2218–30.
34. Oldgren J, Budaj A, Granger CB, et al. Dabigatran vs. placebo in
    patients with acute coronary syndromes on dual antiplatelet
    therapy: a randomized, double-blind, phase II trial. Eur Heart J.
    2011;32:2781–9.
35. Alexander JH, Lopes RD, James S, et al. Apixaban with anti-
    platelet therapy after acute coronary syndrome. N Engl J Med.
    2011;365:699–708.

36. Mega JL, Braunwald E, Wiviott SD, et al. Rivaroxaban in patients with a recent acute coronary syndrome. N Eng J Med. 2011;366:9–19.
37. Andreotti F, Testa L, Biondi-Zoccai GGL, Crea F. Aspirin plus warfarin compared to aspirin alone after acute coronary syndromes: an updated and comprehensive meta-analysis of 25307 patients. Eur Heart J. 2006;27:519–26.
38. Hamm CW, Bassand JP, Agewall S, et al. ESC guidelines for the management of acute coronary syndromes in patients presenting without persistent ST-segment elevation. Eur Heart J. 2011;32: 2999–3054.
39. Writing Group, Wright RS, Anderson JL, et al. 2011 ACCF/ AHA focused update of the guidelines for the management of patients with unstable angina/Non ST-elevation myocardial infarction (updating the 2007 guideline). Circulation. 2011;123: 2022–60.
40. Sandercock PA, Counsell C, Gubitz GJ, Tseng MC. Antiplatelet therapy for acute ischaemic stroke. Cochrane Database Syst Rev. 2008;3:CD000029.
41. National Clinical Guideline for diagnosis and intial management of acute stroke and transient ischaemic attack (TIA). Royal College of Physicians; 2008. ISBN 978-86016-339-5.
42. A national clinical guideline. Management of patients with stroke or TIA: assessment, investigation, immediate management and secondary prevention. Edinburgh: Scottish Intercollegiate Guidelines Network; 2008.
43. Hart RG, Palacio S, Pearce LA. Atrial fibrillation, stroke, and acute antithrombotic therapy. Stroke. 2002;33:2722–7.
44. Hacke W, Kaste M, Bluhmki E, et al. Thrombolysis with alteplase 3 to 4.5 hours after acute ischemic stroke. N Engl J Med. 2008;359: 1317–29.
45. Saver JL. Number needed to treat estimates incorporating effects over the entire range of clinical outcomes: novel derivation method and application to thrombolytic therapy for acute stroke. Arch Neurol. 2004;61:1066–70.
46. Association of Outcome With Early Stroke Treatment. Pooled analysis of ATLANTIS, ECASS, and NINDS Rt-PA stroke trials [abstr]. Lancet. 2004;363:768–74.
47. Wahlgren N, Ahmed N, Dávalos A, et al. Thrombolysis with alteplase for acute ischaemic stroke in the safe implementation of thrombolysis in stroke-monitoring study (SITS-MOST): an observational study [abstr]. Lancet. 2007;369:275–82.

172   J. Watt et al.

48. Nishant KM, Niaz A, Grethe A, et al. Thrombolysis in very elderly people: controlled comparison of SITS international stroke thrombolysis registry and virtual international stroke trials archive. BMJ. 2010;341:c6046.
49. Furlan A, Higashida R, Wechsler L, et al. Intra-arterial prourokinase for acute ischemic stroke. JAMA. 1999;282:2003–11.
50. Farrell B, Godwin J, Richards S, Warlow C. The United Kingdom transient ischaemic attack (UK-TIA) aspirin trial: final results. J Neurol Neurosurg Psychiatry. 1991;54:1044–54.
51. Randomised A. Blinded, trial of clopidogrel versus aspirin in patients at risk of ischaemic events (CAPRIE) [abstr]. Lancet. 1996;348:1329–39.
52. Leonardi-Bee J, Bath PMW, Bousser MG, et al. Dipyridamole for preventing recurrent ischemic stroke and other vascular events. Stroke. 2005;36:162–8.
53. European Stroke Prevention Study. ESPS group. Stroke. 1990; 21:1122–30.
54. Halkes PH. Aspirin plus dipyridamole versus aspirin alone after cerebral ischaemia of arterial origin (ESPRIT): randomised controlled trial [abstr]. Lancet. 2006;367:1665–73.
55. Sacco RL, Diener HC, Yusuf S, et al. Aspirin and extended-release dipyridamole versus clopidogrel for recurrent stroke. N Engl J Med. 2008;359:1238–51.
56. Diener HC, Bogousslavsky J, Brass LM, et al. Aspirin and clopidogrel compared with clopidogrel alone after recent ischaemic stroke or transient ischaemic attack in high-risk patients (MATCH): randomised, double-blind, placebo-controlled trial [abstr]. Lancet. 2004;364:331–7.
57. Bhatt DL, Fox KAA, Hacke W, et al. Clopidogrel and aspirin versus aspirin alone for the prevention of atherothrombotic events. N Engl J Med. 2006;354:1706–17.
58. Atrial Fibrillation Investigators: Atrial Fibrillation AAS, Boston Area Anticoagulation Trial for Atrial Fibrillation Study, Canadian Atrial Fibrillation Anticoagulation Study, Stroke Prevention in Atrial Fibrillation Study, Veterans Affairs Stroke Prevention in Nonrheumatic Atrial Fibrillation Study. Risk factors for stroke and efficacy of antithrombotic therapy in atrial fibrillation: analysis of pooled data from five randomized controlled trials. Arch Intern Med. 1994;154:1449–57.
59. EAFT (European Atrial Fibrillation Trial) Study Group. Secondary prevention in non-rheumatic atrial fibrillation after transient ischaemic attack or minor stroke. Lancet. 1993;342:1255–62.

60. Connolly S, et al. Clopidogrel plus aspirin versus oral anticoagulation for atrial fibrillation in the atrial fibrillation clopidogrel trial with irbesartan for prevention of vascular events (ACTIVE W): a randomised controlled trial [abstr]. Lancet. 2006;367:1903–12.
61. Rothwell PM, Giles MF, Chandratheva A, et al. Effect of urgent treatment of transient ischaemic attack and minor stroke on early recurrent stroke (EXPRESS study): a prospective population-based sequential comparison [abstr]. Lancet. 2007;370:1432–42.

Chapter 5
Approaches to the Prophylaxis and Treatment of Venous and Cardiac Thromboembolic Disease

Christopher Dittus and Jack Ansell

Pathophysiology and Epidemiology of Venous Thromboembolism

Virchow's Triad

Rudolf Virchow, the 19th century German physician, described three factors that contribute to venous thrombosis: (1) Phenomena due to irritation of the vessel and its surroundings; (2) Phenomena due to blood coagulation; and (3) Phenomena due to the interruption of the blood stream [1]. An updated description of these factors is: (1) Alteration in blood flow (i.e. stasis); (2) Vascular endothelial injury; and (3) Hypercoagulability. Clot formation does not require the presence of all factors; however there is an additive risk with increasing factors. Thus, this triad forms the basis for risk factor analysis for venous thromboembolism (VTE).

C. Dittus, D.O., M.P.H. • J. Ansell, M.D.
Department of Medicine, Lenox Hill Hospital,
100 E. 77th Street, New York, NY 10075, USA
e-mail: cdittus@nshs.edu; jansell@nshs.edu

A. Ferro, D.A. Garcia (eds.), *Antiplatelet and Anticoagulation*   175
Therapy, Current Cardiovascular Therapy,
DOI 10.1007/978-1-4471-4297-3_5,
© Springer-Verlag London 2013

Thrombophilia

There are multiple acquired and inherited processes that impart a hypercoagulable state. Acquired hypercoagulable states can be caused by cancer, pregnancy, and hormonal medications (e.g. oral contraceptive pills). Patients may also be hypercoagulable as the result of inherited thrombophilic disorders. There are many thrombophilias – the most important of which are described in Table 5.1. These disorders confer varying risk for thrombus formation. The greatest risk for VTE is in patients with homozygous factor V Leiden with a relative risk of 50–100 fold [2]. Heterozygous factor V Leiden and the prothrombin G20210A gene mutation impart similar, but milder risk for thrombosis, 3–7 and 2–8 fold, respectively. Antithrombin deficiency is associated with fivefold increase in the annual risk of thrombosis. Protein C deficiency is associated with a greater risk of thrombosis than protein S deficiency, 6–10 fold and 2 fold increases, respectively [2]. There is controversy around the testing for hereditary thrombophilias with some studies showing that testing does not predict recurrence after a first episode of VTE [3]. However, this may relate to only some defects, whereas others have a higher likelihood of predicting recurrence [4]. Testing for hereditary thrombophilias may be appropriate in selected circumstances (Table 5.2).

Epidemiology and Characteristics

VTE has a major impact on health in the United States. Some studies suggest that there are more than 900,000 incident and recurrent VTE events annually in the US [5]. Among white Americans, there are at least 250,000 incident cases annually. The incidence in African-Americans is similar or higher than in whites, and in Asian- and Native-Americans the incidence is lower [5]. The risk of VTE is profound in hospitalized patients when compared to those in the community. In one study, the incidence of in-hospital VTE was 960.5 per 10,000 person-years, while the incidence in community residents was 7.1 per 10,000

TABLE 5.1 List of common and uncommon thrombophilias

| Common | Inherited | | Acquired |
	Rare	Very rare	
Factor V Leiden (G1691A mutation)	Antithrombin deficiency	Dysfibrinogenemia	Antiphospholipid syndrome
Prothrombin gene mutation (G20210A)	Protein C deficiency	Homozygous homocystinuria	Heparin-induced Thrombocytopenia (HIT)
	Protein S deficiency		Paroxysmal nocturnal hemoglobinuria (PNH) (rare)

TABLE 5.2 Testing for thrombophilias[a] [84]

Clinical history	Weakly thrombophilic	Strongly thrombophilic
Age at onset <50 year	Negative	Positive
Recurrent thrombosis	Negative	Positive
Family history	Negative	Positive

Adapted from Bauer [84]
[a]Thrombophilia testing is *not* recommended in weakly thrombophilic patients

person-years. [6]. Hospitalization and nursing home residence together account for 60 % of incident VTE events [5].

VTE encompasses two related disease processes: deep venous thrombosis (DVT) and pulmonary embolism (PE) (Fig. 5.1). About two-thirds of VTE episodes manifest as DVT and one-third as PE [7]. Thrombogenesis generally occurs in the deep veins of the lower extremity. Pieces of thrombus can break free from the primary thrombotic lesion and embolize to the right heart via the inferior vena cava. The embolus can then become lodged in the pulmonary vasculature leading to the clinical diagnosis of pulmonary embolism. Many factors contribute to the nature of VTE, and there is a very broad range of clinical pathology. The location of thrombus formation is important clinically because a thrombus in certain locations is associated with a greater risk of embolization. For example, a thrombus in the proximal venous system of the lower extremity is associated with high risk for embolization with half ultimately leading to pulmonary embolism [8]. Thrombus formation in the distal lower extremity is rarely associated with symptomatic PE (<5 %), although asymptomatic PE may be more common (20–30 %) [9]. If untreated, a calf vein thrombus will propagate to the proximal vessels in 25 % of cases, thus leading to an increased risk of embolization [10]. DVT in the upper extremity can also lead to pulmonary embolization, but the emboli tend to be small and less symptomatic.

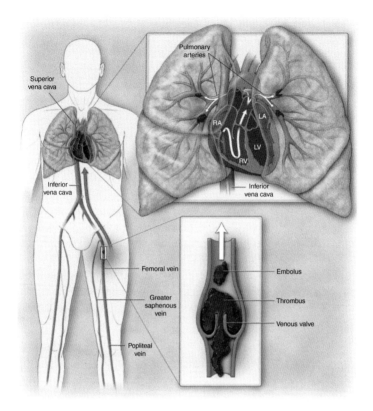

FIGURE 5.1 Pathophysiology of pulmonary embolism (Modified from [88])

Venous Thromboembolism Prevention

Introduction and Risk Factors

VTE is associated with significant morbidity and mortality, with death occurring within 1 month of an episode in 6 % of DVT cases and 10 % of PE cases [7]. The mortality rate for PE is as high as 30 % in studies that include autopsy-diagnosed PE [7]. The 3-month crude mortality rate for PE from the International Pulmonary Embolism Registry was

17.4 % [11]. One-quarter of PE patients have sudden cardiac death as the initial clinical presentation [5]. Morbidity associated with DVT also includes acute pain and swelling of the lower extremity as well as chronic post-thrombotic syndrome and venous ulcer [5]. Furthermore, patients with either DVT or PE are committed to at least 3 months of anticoagulation, which in itself, is associated with inherent risks.

Hospitalized patients have the highest rate of VTE and prophylaxis will be of benefit to many hospitalized patients. However, committing a patient to daily injections of unfractionated heparin (UFH) or low-molecular-weight heparin (LMWH) is not without consequence; therefore the decision to provide DVT prophylaxis must be based on sufficient evidence. The need for VTE prophylaxis in hospitalized patients is based on the fact that VTE is highly prevalent in hospitalized patients, the adverse effects related to VTE are substantial, and effective VTE prophylaxis exists. Defining the group of hospitalized patients who will derive net benefit from mechanical, pharmacologic or combination prophylaxis continues to be a challenge.

Risk Assessment in Medical and Surgical Patients

Current prophylaxis guidelines recommend different prophylaxis regimens in patient populations based on risk of VTE. The major risk factors for DVT can be divided into three categories according to Virchow's triad (see above). Table 5.3 describes the risk factors contributing to each of Virchow's categories. Of note, there is significant overlap between these groups. Additionally, risk factors can be described according to magnitude of risk for VTE (Table 5.4).

The American College of Chest Physicians (ACCP) publishes guidelines on the prevention and treatment of VTE and differentiates hospitalized patients into several groups of varying VTE risk. The most recent guidelines distinguish between nonorthopedic surgical, orthopedic surgery, and nonsurgical patients [12–14]. Surgical patients have an inherent increased risk of VTE relative to nonsurgical patients because

TABLE 5.3 Risk factors for DVT stratified by Virchow's triad

Stasis	Endothelial injury	Hypercoagulability
Surgery	Trauma to lower extremity	Cancer (active or occult)
Immobility/paresis	Vascular surgery	Cancer therapy
Venous compression	Orthopedic surgery	Pregnancy
	Prior DVT	Hormonal treatments (e.g. oral contraceptive pill)
	Central venous catheter	Thrombophilias
		Nephrotic syndrome

TABLE 5.4 Risk factors for DVT stratified by magnitude of risk [9]

Strong risk	Moderate risk	Weak risk
Fracture (hip or leg)	Arthroscopic knee surgery	Bed rest >3 days
Hip/knee replacement	Central venous lines	Immobility due to prolonged sitting
Major general surgery	Chemotherapy	Increasing age
Major trauma	Heart or respiratory failure	Laparoscopic surgery
Spinal cord injury	Hormonal treatments (e.g. oral contraceptive pill)	Obesity
	Malignancy	Pregnancy, antepartum
	Paralytic stroke	Varicose veins
	Pregnancy, postpartum	
	Previous VTE	
	Inherited/acquired thrombophilia	

Adapted from Ansell [9]

of venous stasis during the actual procedure as well as immobility after the intervention. Orthopedic surgery confers an even higher risk of VTE. For example, hip and knee arthroplasty are associated with higher risk of VTE because of direct interaction with the blood vessels in the lower extremity.

VTE risk in nonorthopedic surgery is determined by the patient's baseline risk profile in addition to the type of surgery the patient is undergoing. Baseline risk can be estimated using either the Rogers or Caprini risk assessment models (Tables 5.5 and 5.6) [13, 15–17]. The Rogers model was developed in patients undergoing major general, thoracic or vascular surgery and may be used to risk stratify patients in these surgical groups. The Caprini model has been validated in patients undergoing general surgery, including gastrointestinal, urological, vascular, breast and thyroid procedures [15, 16]. The Caprini model has also been validated in plastic and reconstructive surgery patients. Other surgical populations include spinal surgery, cardiac surgery, thoracic surgery, bariatric surgery, traumatic brain injury and spinal cord injury.

Using the Rogers and Caprini models, surgical patients can be risk-stratified into very low, low, moderate, and high risk for symptomatic VTE [13] (Table 5.7). Surgical populations in which the Rogers and Caprini models have not been validated may be risk-stratified by the type of surgery. Most outpatient surgery are considered very low risk. Spinal surgery for nonmalignant disease is low risk for VTE. Gynecologic noncancer surgery, cardiothoracic surgery, and spinal surgery for malignant disease are considered moderate risk. Bariatric surgery, gynecologic cancer surgery, traumatic brain injury, and spinal cord injury populations are all in the highest risk category. The estimated baseline risk for symptomatic VTE in the absence of prophylaxis for very low risk patients is <0.5 %. For low, moderate, and high risk patients the estimated baseline risk is 1.5, 3, and 6 %, respectively [13].

Patients undergoing major orthopedic surgery, including total hip arthroplasty, total knee arthroplasty, and hip fracture surgery, are at high risk for VTE. Estimated rates for nonfatal, symptomatic VTE in patients not receiving

TABLE 5.5 Risk assessment model from the patient safety in surgery study [17]

Risk factor	Risk score points
Operation type other than endocrine:	
Respiratory and hematological	9
Vascular, incl. thoracoabdominal aneurysm	7
Aneurysm	4
Mouth, palate	4
Stomach, intestines	4
Integument	3
Hernia	2
American Society of Anesthesiologists (ASA) physical status classification:	
3, 4, or 5	2
2	1
Female sex	1
Work relative value unit (RVU):	
>17	3
10–17	2
Two points for each of these conditions:	2
Disseminated cancer	
Chemotherapy for malignancy within 30 d of operation	
Preoperative serum sodium >145 mmol/L	
Transfusion >4 units packed RBCs in 72 h before operation	
Ventilator dependant	
One point for each of these conditions:	1
Wound class (clean/contaminated)	
Preoperative hematocrit level <38 %	
Preoperative bilirubin level >1.0 mg/dL	
Dyspnea	
Albumin level <3.5 mg/dL	
Emergency	
Zero points for each of these conditions:	0
ASA physical status class 1	
Work RVU <10	
Male sex	

Table 5.6 Caprini risk assessment model [13, 15, 16]

1 point	2 points	3 points	5 points
Age 41–60 year	Age 61–74 year	Age >75 year	Stroke (<1 month)
Minor surgery	Arthroscopic surgery	History of VTE	Elective arthroscopy
BMI >25 kg/m^2	Major open surgery (>45 min)	Family history of VTE	Hip, pelvis, or leg fracture
Swollen legs	Laparoscopic surgery (>45 min)	Factor V Leiden	Acute spinal cord injury (<1 month)
Varicose veins	Malignancy	Prothrombin 20210A	
Pregnancy or postpartum	Confined to bed (>72 h)	Lupus anticoagulant	
History of unexplained or recurrent spontaneous abortion	Immobilizing plaster cast	Anticardiolipin antibodies	
Oral contraceptives or hormone replacement	Central venous catheter	Elevated serum homocysteine	
Sepsis (<1 month)		Heparin-induced thrombocytopenia	
Serious lung disease, incl pneumonia (<1 month)		Other congenital or acquired thrombophilia	
Abnormal pulmonary function			
Acute myocardial infarction			
Congestive heart failure (<1 month)			
History of inflammatory bowel disease			
Medical patient at bed rest			

TABLE 5.7 Risk stratification for VTE in non-orthopedic surgical patients and recommended thromboprophylaxis [13]

Risk category for symptomatic VTE (%)	Patients undergoing major general, thoracic, or vascular surgery		Patients undergoing general surgery, including GI, urological, vascular, breast, and thyroid procedures		Patients undergoing plastic and reconstructive surgery		Other surgical populations	Thromboprophylaxis recommendations by VTE risk group and bleeding risk	
	Rogers score	Observed risk of symptomatic VTE, (%)	Caprini score	Observed risk of symptomatic VTE, (%)	Caprini score	Observed risk of VTE, (%)		Average bleeding risk (1 %)	High bleeding risk (2 %) or severe consequences
Very low (<0.5)	<7	0.1	0	0	0–2	NA	Most outpatient or same-day surgery	No specific prophylaxis	
Low (1.5)	7–10	0.4	1–2	0.7	3–4	0.6	Spinal surgery for nonmalignant disease	Mechanical prophylaxis, IPCD preferable	
Moderate (3.0)	≥10	1.5	3–4	1.0	5–6	1.3	Gynecologic noncancer, cardiac, most thoracic, spinal surgery for malignancy	LDUH, LMWH, or mechanical prophylaxis, with IPCD	Mechanical prophylaxis with IPCD

(continued)

186   C. Dittus and J. Ansell

Table 5.7 (continued)

Risk category for symptomatic VTE (%)	Patients undergoing major general, thoracic, or vascular surgery		Patients undergoing general surgery, including GI, urological, vascular, breast, and thyroid procedures		Patients undergoing plastic and reconstructive surgery		Other surgical populations	Thromboprophylaxis recommendations by VTE risk group and bleeding risk	
	Rogers score	Observed risk of symptomatic VTE, (%)	Caprini score	Observed risk of symptomatic VTE, (%)	Caprini score	Observed risk of VTE, (%)		Average bleeding risk (1 %)	High bleeding risk (2 %) or severe consequences
High (6.0)	NA	NA	>5	1.9	7–8	2.7	Bariatric, gynecologic cancer, pneumonectomy, craniotomy, traumatic brain injury, spinal cord injury, other major trauma	LDUH, LMWH, plus mechanical prophylaxis with GCS or IPCD	Mechanical prophylaxis with IPCD, until bleeding risk diminishes and pharmacologic prophylaxis added
High-Risk, LDUH and LMWH contraindicated or unavailable								Fondaparinux or low-dose ASA; mechanical prophylaxis with IPCD; or both	Mechanical prophylaxis with IPCD until bleeding risk diminishes and pharmacologic prophylaxis added

Adapted from Gould et al. [13]

prophylaxis are 2.8 % for postoperative days 0–14 and 1.5 % for days 15–35. The cumulative risk for VTE for postoperative days 0–35 is 4.3 % [12].

The major non-surgical patient groups addressed in the recent ACCP guidelines are hospitalized acutely ill patients and critically ill patients [14]. Hospitalized acutely ill patients have a wide variation in risk for VTE and must be stratified according to a risk assessment model. The best validated of these models is the Padua Prediction Score (Table 5.8), which dichotomizes patients into high- and low-risk categories according to their baseline risk profile [14]. This risk assessment model was studied in a prospective cohort study of over 1,100 patients and found that VTE occurred in 11.0 % of high-risk patients (those with a score greater than or equal to 4) who did not receive thromboprophylaxis and 0.3 % of low-risk patients (those with a score less than 4) [18]. Patients who are high-risk per the Padua Prediction Score should receive thromboprophylaxis. Those who are low-risk should not receive thromboprophylaxis [14]. Critically ill patients are often at increased risk for VTE because of the severity of their disease, but not all critically ill patients have the same baseline risk profile. Unfortunately, there are no validated risk assessment models to stratify critically ill patients by VTE risk (see Fig. 5.2 for an overview of VTE prophylaxis in surgical and nonsurgical patients).

A recent systematic review evaluated the effect of thromboprophylaxis in medical and stroke patients [19]. In this review, heparin prophylaxis did not reduce total mortality in medical patients, but did result in a decreased incidence of pulmonary embolism [19]. Heparin prophylaxis was also found to significantly increase the risk of all bleeding in this group. In patients with acute stroke, heparin prophylaxis had no significant effect on any outcome, but was associated with a statistically significant increase in major bleeding events [19]. The type of heparin used (UFH or LMWH) had no effect on outcome or harms. Prophylaxis with graduated compression stockings had no clinical benefit, but did cause significant lower extremity skin damage in patients with acute stroke [19]. These

TABLE 5.8 Padua prediction score [18]

Risk factor	Points
Active cancer	3
Previous VTE (excluding superficial vein thrombosis)	3
Reduced mobility	3
Already known thrombophilic condition	3
Recent (<1 month) trauma and/or surgery	2
Elderly age (>70 year)	1
Heart and/or respiratory failure	1
Acute myocardial infarction or ischemic stroke	1
Acute infection and/or rheumatologic disorder	1
Obesity (BMI >30)	1
Ongoing hormonal treatment	1

findings led the American College of Physicians (ACP) to publish guidelines recommending: (1) Assessment of risk for VTE and bleeding in medical patients prior to initiating prophylaxis; (2) Heparin or a related drug should be used unless the risk of bleeding outweighs the benefit of prophylaxis; and (3) Against the use of graduated compression stockings [20].

The use of LMWH for VTE prophylaxis in acutely ill medical patients was not associated with a reduction in the rate of death from any cause in a recent randomized trial [21]. The study population included patients with acute decompensated heart failure, severe systemic infection with at least one risk factor for VTE, or those with active cancer. The trial randomized 8,307 participants into a treatment arm receiving enoxaparin 40 mg daily plus elastic stockings with graduated compression and a placebo arm that only receiving elastic stockings with graduated compression. The rate of death at day 30 was 4.9 % in the enoxaparin group and 4.8 % in the placebo group, with a relative risk of 1.0 (CI, 0.8–1.2).

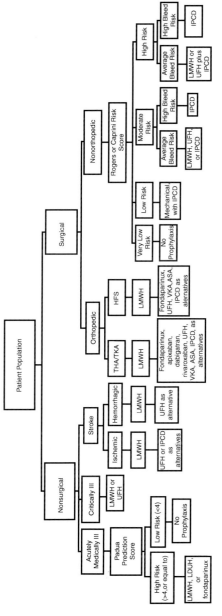

FIGURE 5.2 VTE prophylaxis, summary flowchart. *ASA* aspirin, *IPCD* intermittent pneumatic compression device, *LMWH* low molecular weight heparin, *LDUH/UFH* low-dose/unfractionated heparin, *VKA* vitamin K antagonist, *VTE* venous thromboembolism

Prophylaxis Methods: Medicinal and Non-Medicinal

There are two distinct modalities that can be employed to prevent the formation of DVT: pharmacologic and non-pharmacologic. Pharmacologic prophylaxis includes administration of the following anticoagulants at prophylactic doses: subcutaneous UFH, LMWH, fondaparinux, vitamin K antagonists (VKA), as well as newer oral anticoagulants (direct thrombin inhibitors and activated factor X inhibitors). Non-pharmacologic interventions include graduated compression stockings (GCS), intermittent pneumatic compression devices (IPCD), and early ambulation (Table 5.9).

Nonorthopedic surgery patients must first be stratified by risk to either very-low, low, moderate, or high-risk groups (Table 5.7). This is accomplished by using either the Rogers or Caprini risk assessment models [13] (Tables 5.5, 5.6, and 5.7). Very-low risk patients do not need pharmacologic or mechanical VTE prophylaxis. Low risk patients should receive mechanical VTE prophylaxis with an IPCD. Moderate risk patients with an average bleeding risk should receive LMWH, low-dose UFH, or an IPCD. If the patient has a high risk of bleeding, an IPCD should be used instead of pharmacologic VTE prophylaxis. Patients with high risk of VTE and an average bleeding risk should receive either LMWH, low-dose UFH, plus an IPCD [13]. If the high risk patient is having surgery for cancer, then LMWH should be continued for 4 weeks after discharge [13]. High VTE risk patients who have a high risk of bleeding should use an IPCD.

Orthopedic surgery patients receiving total hip arthroplasty or total knee arthroplasty should receive LMWH, fondaparinux, apixaban, dabigatran, rivaroxaban, low-dose UFH, VKA, ASA or IPCD for 10–14 days after the procedure [12]. LMWH should be used preferentially over the other options. If the patient declines injections, then apixaban or dabigatran should be used over the other oral alternatives. Current guidelines also suggest an extended 35 day course of prophylaxis over the shorter

TABLE 5.9 Methods of VTE prophylaxis

Pharmacologic	Non-pharmacologic
Unfractionated heparin (subcutaneous)	Early ambulation
Low molecular weight heparin	Graduated compression stockings
Factor Xa inhibitors (parenteral and oral)	Intermittent pneumatic compression device
Direct thrombin (factor IIa) inhibitors (parenteral and oral)	
Vitamin K antagonists	
Aspirin	

10–14 day course [12]. An IPCD should be used in addition to pharmacologic prophylaxis whenever possible. The above guidelines apply to hip fracture surgery, except the new oral anticoagulants (apixaban, dabigatran, and rivaroxaban) are not included as prophylaxis alternatives. The section below includes more information on these new agents.

Nonsurgical patients vastly vary in both severity and type of disease. Acutely ill medical patients must be stratified using a risk assessment model, in this case the Padua Prediction Score (Table 5.8). High risk patients should receive LMWH, low-dose UFH (either BID or TID), or fondaparinux [14]. If the patient is at high risk for bleeding, then either GCS or an IPCD should be used. Guidelines suggest against an extended course of VTE prophylaxis beyond the period of immobilization or hospitalization [14]. Low risk patients should not receive VTE prophylaxis. Critically ill patients should receive LMWH or low-dose UFH for VTE prophylaxis [14]. If the patient has a high-risk of bleeding, then GCS or an IPCD should be used. Patients with acute ischemic stroke and restricted mobility should receive LMWH, low-dose UFH, or an IPCD [22]. Patients with acute primary intracerebral hemorrhage and restricted mobility should receive LMWH or low-dose UFH starting 2–4 days after the event, or an IPCD [22]. For either type of stroke, LMWH should be used preferentially over either low-dose UFH or an IPCD. Guidelines suggest against using GCS's. Outpatients with cancer and no other risk factors for VTE should not receive VTE prophylaxis [14]. Outpatients with cancer and another risk factor for VTE should receive LMWH or low-dose UFH.

New Oral Anticoagulants

Direct thrombin and factor Xa inhibitors are being extensively studied for the prevention of thromboembolic stroke in patients with atrial fibrillation, for primary and secondary prevention of VTE, and for prevention of recurrent myocardial infarction in patients with acute coronary syndrome. The new anticoagulant agents are grouped into two classes based on the clotting factor that is inhibited in the clotting cascade (factor Xa or factor IIa). The factor Xa inhibitors bind directly to the enzymatic pocket of factor Xa and inhibit its function in the prothrombinase complex thus limiting thrombin generation. The factor IIa (thrombin) inhibitors act by directly binding to the enzymatic pocket of thrombin and preventing the conversion of fibrinogen to fibrin as well as the activation of platelets. These agents have potential advantages over the VKAs in that they do not require monitoring, they have very few significant drug interactions, and they have a rapid onset and offset of action (see Chapter 3 for more detail).

For VTE prophylaxis in major orthopedic surgery, dabigatran etexilate, a direct thrombin inhibitor, was shown to be comparable to enoxaparin 40 mg daily [23, 24], but when compared to enoxaparin 30 mg twice daily, it fell short of meeting the non-inferiority criteria for the trial [25] (Table 5.10). Apixaban, a direct factor Xa inhibitor was superior to enoxaparin 40 mg daily [26, 27], but just failed to meet the non-inferiority criteria when compared to enoxaparin 30 mg twice daily [28] (Table 5.10). Rivaroxaban, another direct factor Xa inhibitor, was shown to be superior to enoxaparin in major orthopedic surgery, using either dosing scheme for enoxaparin [29–31] (Table 5.10).

TABLE 5.10 Comparison of trials evaluating dabigatran, rivaroxaban, and apixaban for VTE prophylaxis after orthopedic surgery

Study	Drug, dose	Number, duration	Indication	Comparator	Primary outcome measure	Primary safety measure	Primary outcome results	Primary safety results
RE-MOBILIZE [25]	Dabigatran 150 or 220 mg daily	2,615, 12–15 days	TKR	Enoxaparin 30 mg BID	Total VTE and all-cause mortality	Major bleeding	150 mg: 34 %, 219/649, RD: 8.4 % (CI: 3.4–13.3)	150 mg: 0.6 %, 5/871
							220 mg: 31 %, 188/604, RD:5.8 % (CI:0.8–10.8)	220 mg: 0.6, 5/857
							Enox: 25 %, 163/643	Enox: 1.4 %, 12/868
							Dabigatran not *noninferior*	*No increase in major bleeding with either dabigatran dosing*

(continued)

TABLE 5.10 (continued)

Study	Drug, dose	Number, duration	Indication	Comparator	Primary outcome measure	Primary safety measure	Primary outcome results	Primary safety results
RE-MODEL [29]	Dabigatran 150 or 220 mg daily	2,076, 6–10 days	TKR	Enoxaparin 40 mg daily	Total VTE and all-cause mortality	Major bleeding	150 mg: 40.5 %, 213/526, AD: 1.3 % (CI: 7.3–4.6)	150 mg: 1.3 %, 9/703
							220 mg: 36.4 %, 183/503, AD: 2.8 % (CI: 3.1–8.7)	220 mg: 1.5 %, 10/679
							Enox: 37.7 %, 193/512	Enox: 1.3 %, 9/694
							Dabigatran noninferior	*No increase in major bleeding with either dabigatran dosing*

Study	Drug	N, duration	Procedure	Comparator	Primary outcome	Secondary outcome	Efficacy	Safety
RE-NOVATE [23, 24]	Dabigatran 150 or 220 mg daily	3,494, 28–35 days	THR	Enoxaparin 40 mg daily	Total VTE and all-cause mortality	Major bleeding	150 mg: 8.6 %, 75/874, AD:1.9 (CI: 0.6–4.4); 220 mg: 6 %, 53/880, AD: 0.7 (CI: 2.9–1.6); Enox: 6.7 %, 60/897; *Dabigatran noninferior*	150 mg: 1.3 %, 15/1,163; 220 mg: 2 %, 23/1,146; Enox: 1.6 %, 18/1,154; *No increase in major bleeding with either dabigatran dosing*
RE-NOVATE II [85]	Dabigatran 220 mg daily	2,055, 28–35 days	THR	Enoxaparin 40 mg daily	Composite of VTE and all-cause mortality	Major bleeding	Dab: 7.7 %, 61/792; Enox: 8.8 %, 69/785, RD: 1.1 (CI: 3.8–1.6); *Dabigatran noninferior*	Dab: 1.4 %, 14/1,010; Enox: 0.9 %, 9/1,003; *No increase in major bleeding with dabigatran*

(continued)

TABLE 5.10 (continued)

Study	Drug, dose	Number, duration	Indication	Comparator	Primary outcome measure	Primary safety measure	Primary outcome results	Primary safety results
ADVANCE-1 [28]	Apixaban 2.5 mg BID	3,195, 12 days	TKR	Enoxaparin 30 mg BID	Composite VTE and all-cause mortality	Major bleeding	Apix: 9 %, 104/1,157 Enox: 8.8 %, 100/1,130, RR: 1.02 (CI: 0.78–1.32) *Apixaban not noninferior*	Apix: 0.7 %, 11/1,596 Enox: 1.4 %, 22/1,588, ADJ: 0.81 (CI: 1.49–0.14) *No increase in major bleeding.*
ADVANCE-2 [26, 27]	Apixaban 2.5 mg BID	1,973, 12 days	TKR	Enoxaparin 40 mg daily	Composite VTE and all-cause mortality	Major bleeding	Apix: 15 %, 147/976 Enox: 24 %, 243/997, RR: 0.62 (CI: 0.51–0.74) *Apixaban superior*	Apix: 0.6 %, 9/1,501 Enox: 0.9 %, 14/1,508, AD: 0.33 (CI: 0.95–0.29) *No increase in major bleeding with apixaban*

Study	Drug	N, days	Setting	Comparator	Efficacy outcome	Efficacy result	Safety outcome	Safety result
ADVANCE-3 [26, 27]	Apixaban 2.5 mg BID	5,407, 35 days	THR	Enoxaparin 40 mg daily	Composite VTE and all-cause mortality	Apix: 1.4 %, 27/1,949 Enox: 3.9 %, 74/1,917, RR: 0.36 (CI: 0.22–0.54) *Apixaban superior*	Major bleeding	Apix: 0.8 %, 22/2,673 Enox: 0.7 %, 18/2,659, AD: 0.2 (CI: 1.4–1) *No increase in major bleeding with apixaban*
RECORD-1 [29]	Rivaroxaban 10 mg daily	4,541, 35 days	THR	Enoxaparin 40 mg daily	Composite VTE and all-cause mortality	Riv: 1.1 %, 18/1,595 Enox: 3.7 %, 58/1,558, AR: 2.6 (CI: 1.5–3.7) *Rivaroxaban superior*	Major bleeding	Riv: 0.3 %, 6/2,209 Enox: 0.1 %, 2/2,224 *p-value: 0.18, no increase in major bleeding*
RECORD-2 [86]	Rivaroxaban 10 mg daily	2,509, 31–39 days	THR	Enoxaparin 40 mg daily (10–14 days)	Composite VTE and all-cause mortality	Riv: 2 %, 17/864 Enox: 9.3 %, 81/869, AR: 7.3 (CI: 2–9.4) *Rivaroxaban superior*	Major bleeding	Riv: <0.1 %, 1/1,228 Enox: <0.1 %, 1/1,229 *p-value: 0.25, no increase in major bleeding*

(continued)

TABLE 5.10 (continued)

Study	Drug, dose	Number, duration	Indication	Comparator	Primary outcome measure	Primary safety measure	Primary outcome results	Primary safety results
RECORD-3 [30]	Rivaroxaban 10 mg daily	2,531, 10–14 days	TKR	Enoxaparin 40 mg daily	Composite VTE and all-cause mortality	Major bleeding	Riv: 9.6 %, 79/824 Enox: 18.9 %, 166/878, AR: 9.2 (CI:5.9–12.4) *Rivaroxaban superior*	Riv: 0.6 %, 7/1,220 Enox: 0.5 %, 6/1,239, AR: 0.1(p=0.77) *No increase in major bleeding*
RECORD-4 [31]	Rivaroxaban 10 mg daily	3,148, 10–14 days	TKR	Enoxaparin 30 mg BID	Composite VTE and all-cause mortality	Major bleeding	Riv: 6.9 %, 67/965 Enox: 10.1 %, 97/959, AR: 3.19 (CI: 0.71–5.67) *Rivaroxaban superior*	Riv: 0.7 %, 10/1,526 Enox: 0.3 %, 4/1,508 *p-value: 0.1096, no increase in major bleeding*

AD absolute risk difference, *ADJ* adjusted risk difference, *AR* absolute risk reduction *apix* apixaban, *CI* confidence interval, *Dab* dabigatran, *Enox* enoxaparin, *RD* risk difference, *Riv* rivaroxaban, *RR* relative risk, *THR* total hip replacement, *TKR* total knee replacement, *VTE* venous thromboembolism

Rivaroxaban is currently approved for DVT prophylaxis in major orthopedic surgery in the United States.

Rivaroxaban and apixaban have both been studied as DVT prophylaxis in medically ill hospitalized patients with extended therapy for approximately 30 days post-discharge [32, 33]. Neither drug resulted in a benefit compared to enoxaparin during the inpatient phase of the studies. During the post-discharge phase, rivaroxaban showed a significant reduction in VTE, but a significant increase in major bleeding that outweighed the benefit [32]. Apixaban failed to show a significant reduction in VTE and resulted in a mild increase in major bleeding [33] (Table 5.11).

Another group of medications, the HMG CoA reductase inhibitors (statins), have been studied regarding their utility in preventing VTE on a long-term basis. The JUPITER study, a large, randomized, double-blind, placebo-controlled trial, evaluated rosuvastatin in the prevention of VTE in men >50 and women >60 with no history of cardiovascular disease, LDL < 130, and high-sensitivity CRP > 2. This study found that rosuvastatin significantly reduced symptomatic VTE in otherwise healthy individuals [34]. However, this therapy has not been studied for the immediate, short-term prevention of VTE in patients at risk.

Venous Thromboembolism Diagnosis and Treatment

Diagnosis, Risk Scores, Tests

Making an accurate diagnosis in a timely fashion is of the utmost importance given the significant morbidity and mortality associated with VTE. The clinical presentation of DVT overlaps with several other disease processes affecting the lower extremity including edema related to heart failure, cellulitis, muscle strain, and trauma. Through the history and physical examination, the diagnosis can often be suspected, but this is not sufficient and the diagnosis of DVT must be made through objective, confirmatory imaging studies.

Table 5.11 Comparison of trials evaluating rivaroxaban and apixaban for VTE prophylaxis in medically ill patients

Study	Drug, dose	Number, duration	Indication	Comparator	Primary outcome measure	Primary safety measure	Primary outcome results	Primary safety results
ADOPT [33]	Apixaban 2.5 mg BID	6,528, 30 days	VTE prophylaxis in medically ill patients	Enoxaparin 40 mg daily (6–14 days)	30-day composite of death related to VTE, PE, DVT	Major bleeding	Apix: 2.71 %, 60/2,211 Enox: 3.06 %, 70/2,284, RR: 0.87 (CI: 0.62–1.23) *Apixaban not superior to enoxaparin*	Apix: 0.47 %, 15/3,184 Enox: 0.19 %, 6/3,217, RR: 2.58 (CI: 1.02–7.24) *Apixaban had increased major bleeding*

Study	Drug	N, duration	Indication	Comparator	Composite of VTE-related death, PE, DVT	Major bleeding and clinically relevant nonmajor bleeding	Efficacy results	Safety results
MAGELLAN [32]	Rivaroxaban 10 mg daily	8,100, 35 days	VTE prophylaxis in medically ill patients	Enoxaparin 40 mg daily (10 days)	Composite of VTE-related death, PE, DVT	Major bleeding and clinically relevant nonmajor bleeding	Day 10: Riv: 2.7 %, 79/2939 Enox: 2.7 %, 80/2993, HR: 0.968 (CI: 0.71–1.33) Day 35: Riv: 4.4 %, 130/2967 Enox: 5.7 %, 174/3,057, HR: 0.77 (CI: 0.62–0.96) *Rivaroxaban noninferior at day 10, superior at day 35.*	Day 10: Riv: 2.8 %, 111/3997 Enox: 1.2 %, 48/4001, HR: 2.3(p = <0.0001) Day 35: Riv: 4.2 %, 167/3997 Enox: 1.7 %, 68/4,001, HR: 3(p = <0.0001) *Rivaroxaban had increased clinically significant bleeding*

Apix apixaban, *CI* confidence interval, *Enox* enoxaparin, *HR* Hazard ratio, *Riv* rivaroxaban, *RR* relative risk, *VTE* venous thromboembolism

Common presenting signs and symptoms include lower extremity swelling, erythema, and calf tenderness on palpation (Homan's Sign). For many patients, the pre-test probabliltiy of DVT can be quantified using a clinical prediction rule such as the Wells Score [35, 36] (Table 5.12).

TABLE 5.12 Wells score for pre-test probability in patients with suspected DVT [35, 36]

Parameter	Points
Historical	
Active cancer	+1
Bedridden >3 days or major surgery within 4 weeks	+1
Paralysis, paresis, recent immobilization of lower extremity	+1
Previous DVT	+1
Alternative diagnosis to DVT as/more likely	–2
Physical exam	
Calf Swelling >3 cm compared to other leg	+1
Dilated superficial collateral veins	+1
Entire leg swollen	+1
Tenderness along deep venous system	+1
Pitting edema greater in symptomatic leg	+1

Traditional score [35]:

3–8 points: high probability of DVT (53/71, 74.6 % CI: 63–84)

1–2 points: moderate probability of DVT (32/193, 16.6 % CI: 12–23)

–2 to 0 points: low probability of DVT (10/329, 3 % CI: 1.7–5.9)

Dichotomized score [36]:

2 or more points: DVT likely (138/495, 27.5 % CI: 23.9–31.8)

Less than 2 points: DVT unlikely (32/587, 5.5 % CI: 3.8–7.6)

DVT deep vein thrombosis

Once a score has been calculated, the clinician uses the risk prediction model to guide the patient's management. When using a dichotomized risk prediction model [36], a patient with a low-risk score and hence a low pre-test probability, can be further evaluated with a sensitive (95–99 %) D-dimer assay taken from the peripheral blood [37, 38]. If the D-dimer concentration is <500 ng/ml, DVT can be ruled-out as a possible diagnosis. If the D-dimer concentration is >500 ng/ml then an imaging modality must be pursued because the D-dimer concentration has a low specificity (32–46 %) [37, 38]. The "gold standard" diagnostic test is venography, but this is rarely used given the excellent sensitivity (96 %) and specificity (98 %) of ultrasound imaging with compression ultrasonography, which is far less expensive and invasive [39]. A high pre-test probability warrants investigation with ultrasound imaging, without first obtaining a D-dimer level.

When using a traditional risk prediction model with low, moderate, and high pre-test probabilities [35], a patient with a moderate pre-test probability can have a DVT ruled out only with a *highly*-sensitive D-dimer assay, otherwise the patient must have ultrasound imaging with Doppler [40]. A patient with a low pre-test probability can have a DVT ruled out with a *moderate or high* sensitivity D-dimer assay [40]. As above, a patient with a high pre-test probability for DVT must have ultrasound imaging with Doppler [40].

The clinical approach to PE is similar to that for DVT. The typical clinical presentation of PE includes symptoms such as dyspnea and chest pain. Common signs are tachycardia and tachypnea. Chest radiography may reveal the Westermark sign (an abrupt cutoff of pulmonary vascularity distal to a large central pulmonary embolus) or Hampton's hump (a shallow wedge-shaped opacity in the periphery of the lung with its base against the pleural surface). The differential diagnosis is broad for dyspnea and/or chest pain; therefore the clinician must have a high clinical suspicion for PE. Once PE has been included in the differential diagnosis, a pre-test probability can be calculated [41–44] (Table 5.13).

TABLE 5.13 Wells prediction rule for patients with suspected PE [41–43]

Parameter	Points
Historical	
PE is #1 diagnosis, or equally likely	+3
Immobilization >3 days or Surgery within 4 weeks	+1.5
Prior PE or DVT	+1.5
Hemoptysis	+1
Malignancy (treatment within 6 months or palliative)	+1
Physical Exam	
Clinical signs and symptoms of DVT	+3
Heart rate over 100	+1.5

Traditional score, use with V/Q [42, 43]:

>6 points: high probability of PE (24/64, 40.6 % CI: 28.7–53.7)

2–6 points: moderate probability of PE (55/339, 16.2 % CI: 12.5–20.6)

<2 points: low probability of PE (7/527, 1.3 % CI: 0.5–2.7)

Dichotomized score, use with CTA [41, 42]:

Greater than 4 points: PE likely (408/1,100, 37.1 % (CI: 34.2–40))

Less than or equal to 4 points: PE unlikely (266/2,206, 12.1 % CI: 1.7–13.5)

CTA Computed tomography angiography, *DVT* deep vein thrombosis, *PE* pulmonary embolism, *V/Q* ventilation perfusion scan

In a patient with an "unlikely" dichotomized Wells score, and thus a low pre-test probability, PE can be excluded with a D-dimer <500 ng/ml [41, 42]. If the D-dimer is >500 ng/ml in a patient with a low pre-test probability, an imaging modality must be pursued. In patients with a high Wells score, and thus a high pre-test probability, an imaging modality must be pursued regardless of D-dimer concentration [41, 43]. Pulmonary angiography, the historic gold standard for PE, has been replaced by CT Angiography which has good sensitivity

(83 %) and excellent specificity (96 %) for PE [39]. The addition of venous-phase CT venography has increased the sensitivity of CTA to 90 % [45]. With a high pre-test probability, the positive predictive value (PPV) of CTA for diagnosing PE is 96 % [39]. CTA requires IV contrast and therefore, patients with renal insufficiency or contrast allergy must have alternative diagnostic imaging, such as ventilation-perfusion scanning. This modality has excellent sensitivity (98 %), but lacks specificity (10 %) [46]. A high-probability ventilation-perfusion scan requires two or more segmental perfusion defects in the presence of *normal* ventilation. Unfortunately, many scans have an abnormal ventilation component, which can be caused by preexisting lung pathology, and the resulting scan is nondiagnostic [33]. If this imaging modality is pursued, a traditional risk prediction model must be used that stratifies patients into low, moderate, and high pre-test probability [43]. Patients with a moderate or high pre-test probability must receive imaging, whereas those with a low pre-test probability can have PE ruled out with a negative D-dimer assay [43].

If the patient is presenting with hemodynamic instability, is critically ill, and if there is a high clinical suspicion for PE, transthoracic or transesophageal echocardiology should be pursued. If there is no right ventricular dysfunction in the setting of hemodynamic instability, the clinician must pursue an alternate diagnosis. If there is right ventricular dysfunction, in the setting of hemodynamic instability and high suspicion for PE, PE is confirmed [47].

Initial Treatment

The initial treatment of proximal lower extremity DVT involves the use of a rapidly acting anticoagulant along with the early initiation of a VKA (e.g. warfarin). Guidelines from the ACCP recommend the use of LMWH, fondaparinux, IV UFH, or SC UFH for parenteral anticoagulation [48]. LMWH or fondaparinux are suggested over IV or SC UFH [48]. Parenteral anticoagulation should be continued for at least 5 days while awaiting the VKA to reach therapeutic levels

(INR target 2–3) and the patient must have a therapeutic INR for >24 h before stopping parenteral anticoagulation. Alternatively, the most recent ACCP guidelines also recommend rivaroxaban for initial treatment of VTE, although this medication is not FDA-approved for this indication [48]. If this treatment option is pursued, no parenteral anticoagulation is indicated. Patients with high or intermediate clinical suspicion for DVT should be started on parenteral anticoagulation prior to full diagnostic workup [48]. Patients with low clinical suspicion can await full diagnostic testing prior to initiating anticoagulation. Invasive modalities are currently being studied that directly dissolve or remove the thrombus. These modalities include catheter-directed thrombolysis (CDT), systemic thrombolysis, and operative venous thrombectomy. An ongoing, phase III, randomized, controlled trial, the ATTRACT study, is assessing the efficacy of CDT at preventing post-thrombotic syndrome (PTS) [49]. In this trial 692 patients with symptomatic proximal DVT will be randomized to receive CDT plus anticoagulation and GCS or anticoagulation and GCS alone. In the future, this approach may be warranted in certain patients at high-risk of PTS, but current guidelines suggest anticoagulant therapy alone for most patients [48].

In patients who have acute proximal DVT of the lower extremity and a contraindication to anticoagulation, an inferior vena cava (IVC) filter should be placed [48]. If the bleeding risk resolves, the patient should receive a full course of anticoagulation.

Distal DVT of the lower extremity can receive a brief (6–12 week) course of anticoagulation. If the patient presents without severe symptoms, he or she can receive serial imaging to evaluate for extension of the thrombus. If the thrombus does not extend further, anticoagulation can be avoided. If the thrombus extends proximally, the patient should receive a full course of anticoagulation and should be managed in the same manner as an initial proximal DVT [48].

Patients with superficial vein thrombosis of the lower limb can be managed conservatively (NSAIDs + warm compresses) or receive a prophylactic dose of fondaparinux or LMWH for 45 days if the thrombus is at least 5 cm in length [48].

Patients with upper extremity thrombosis in the axillary vein, or more proximal, should receive acute, parenteral anticoagulation with LMWH, fondaparinux, or UFH (IV or SC) [48]. LMWH or fondaparinux are preferred over UFH. Patients with upper extremity DVT should be anticoagulated for a minimum of 3 months. If the patient has a central venous catheter (CVC) that is not removed, then anticoagulation should be continued as long as the CVC remains inserted [48].

The acute treatment of PE is more complicated than the acute treatment of DVT because the patient's hemodynamic stability must be evaluated. Acute PE can be divided into three categories of severity – massive, submassive, and nonmassive (Table 5.14). Massive PE is defined as shock or sustained hypotension (SBP < 90 mmHg or a pressure drop of >40 mmHg for >15 min) in the setting of confirmed PE. Hemodynamically stable patients with PE can be divided into submassive and nonmassive based on the presence of right ventricular dysfunction and/or injury. Those without RV dysfunction or injury are deemed nonmassive; those with dysfunction and/or injury are categorized as submassive. The submassive category can be further divided into those with RV dysfunction (abnormal RV imaging) alone and those with dysfunction and injury (abnormal cardiac biomarkers). Patients with both dysfunction and injury have a worse prognosis [47].

Treatment of acute PE is determined by risk-stratifying the patient. A patient with massive PE requires emergent life-saving intervention. The ACCP suggests short-course thrombolytic therapy for patients with massive PE [48]. The American Heart Association (AHA) has published recommendations for the management of massive and submassive PE stating that thrombolysis is a reasonable approach for massive PE [50]. Thrombolysis may also be considered in submassive PE with severe cardiac dysfunction and injury [50]. The ACCP suggests systemic thrombolysis be administered to patients with submassive PE who are at high risk of developing hypotension [48]. Most physicians would agree that the risks of thrombolysis outweigh the benefits in

TABLE 5.14 Acute pulmonary embolism risk stratification

| Parameter | Nonmassive PE | Submassive PE | | Massive PE |
		Dysfunction alone	Dysfunction + injury	
nonmassive PE (echo and/or CTA)	Normal	Abnormal	Abnormal	Abnormal
Cardiac biomarkers(NT-BNP, troponin)	Normal	Normal	Abnormal	Abnormal
Hemodynamics (blood pressure)	Normal	Normal	Normal	Abnormal

CTA Computed tomography angiography, *Echo* Echocardiogram, *NT-BNP* N-terminal fragment, brain natriuretic peptide, *PE* pulmonary embolism, *RV* right ventricle (of the heart)

patients with submassive PE with RV dysfunction but no injury, although this view is not supported by sufficient evidence. The AHA recommends against thrombolysis in nonmassive PE as well as submassive acute PE with minor RV dysfunction or injury [50]. Another intervention for massive PE is thrombectomy, which can be achieved via percutaneous catheterization or an open procedure [50]. Either approach is reasonable if there is a contraindication to thrombolysis, or if it is not available in a given institution [50]. Further, if a patient with massive PE remains hemodynamically unstable after thrombolysis, thrombectomy is a reasonable second-line approach [50]. The ACCP has similar recommendations, reserving catheter-directed thrombectomy as an alternative if there is a contraindication to, or if the patient failed, thrombolysis [48]. Surgical pulmonary thrombectomy should be pursued only if thrombolysis and catheter-directed thrombolysis have failed or are contraindicated [48]. The only anticoagulant that has been evaluated for use with thrombolytic therapy is intravenous unfractionated heparin. Therefore initial anticoagulation should be with intravenous unfractionated heparin in any patient being considered for thrombolysis [47]. In patients with high or intermediate clinical suspicion for PE, anticoagulant treatment should be initiated while awaiting the results of confirmatory testing [48]. In patients with low clinical suspicion, physicians may await results of diagnostic imaging.

Acute treatment of nonmassive and submassive PE involves the use of an immediately acting anticoagulant. Current guidelines from the ACCP recommend the use of either LMWH, fondaparinux, or UFH (IV or SC) [48]. LMWH or fondaparinux are suggested over IV or SC UFH [48]. Rivaroxaban may also be used for the initial treatment of PE, although this medication is not currently FDA-approved for this indication [48]. Patients with acute PE may be treated outside the hospital if they have a reliable home support system, are clinically stable, lack chest pain or dyspnea, have normal right ventricle size and function, and normal levels of cardiac biomarkers [33, 48]. Patients presenting with a pulmonary embolism severity index of risk class I or II can be safely treated in the outpatient setting according to a recently published study [51].

Current guidelines recommend that patients with PE receive LMWH, UFH, or fondaparinux for at least 5 days while bridging to a VKA [48]. The VKA should be initiated on the first treatment day and the LMWH, UFH, or fondaparinux should be continued until the INR is >2 for at least 24 h [48]. If a patient has a contraindication to anticoagulation, an inferior vena cava (IVC) filter must be inserted [48]. When the patient's risk of bleeding resolves, the patient should receive a full course of anticoagulation, and, if feasible, the IVC filter should be removed.

Chronic Treatment of VTE

When it is determined that a patient is clinically stable, the remainder of the therapy can occur in the outpatient setting. Chronic treatment of VTE traditionally involves the use of long-term oral VKA therapy after a bridge from a rapidly acting, parenteral anticoagulant (see above). The patient must be transitioned from a rapidly acting anticoagulant to a VKA because of the VKA's delayed onset of action, relating to clotting factor half-life. The vitamin K dependent clotting factors are II, VII, IX, X, Protein C and Protein S. Factor II has the longest half-life, 60 h, and is primarily responsible for the delayed anticoagulant effect of VKA therapy.

The ACCP suggests a VKA be used for chronic treatment of VTE, with a target INR of 2–3 [48]. If an alternative to a VKA is used, the ACCP suggests LMWH over dabigatran or rivaroxaban [48]. In a limited number of circumstances it is advisable to use LMWH instead of a VKA. Guidelines [48] currently suggest the use of LMWH in patients with active cancer based on the study by Lee et al. [52] showing a significant reduction in recurrence compared with VKA treatment. If an alternative to LMWH is used, guidelines suggest a VKA be used over dabigatran or rivaroxaban [48]. New oral medications serving as alternatives to warfarin therapy will be discussed further at the end of this section.

Duration of Treatment for VTE

Treatment duration for all patients with an initial VTE is at least 3 months [48]. The continuation of anticoagulation therapy is then determined by the patient's initial risk factors. If the patient has a provoked but *reversible* risk factor (also called "secondary VTE") (Table 5.15) such as recent surgery, then the treatment duration may be limited to 3 months [48]. If the patient has a provoked but *irreversible* risk factor, or if the VTE is unprovoked (also called "idiopathic VTE"), then the patient should receive 3 months of anticoagulation and then be evaluated for the risk versus benefit of extended anticoagulation beyond 3 months [48]. The ACCP currently suggests extended anticoagulation for patients with unprovoked VTE and low or moderate bleeding risk [48]. For those patients with high bleeding risk, anticoagulation should be limited to 3 months [48]. Compared to those with provoked VTE, patients with idiopathic VTE have a high risk for recurrence after anticoagulant therapy is discontinued.

TABLE 5.15 Classification of VTE risk factors to guide duration of therapy

Provoked and reversible (secondary)	Provoked and irreversible	Unprovoked
Surgery	Ongoing cancer	Prolonged travel
Hospitalization	Long-term immobility	Idiopathic
Plaster cast immobilization	Selected thrombophilias	
Hormonal treatment		
Pregnancy		
Trauma		
Indwelling catheter		

VTE venous thromboembolism

Risk Assessment for Recurrence

When evaluating a patient for recurrence of VTE, the patient's initial risk factors must be revisited. If the patient had a reversible, provoked risk factor, then the likelihood of recurrent VTE is low. This is reflected in treatment guidelines as these patients will only receive 3 months of anticoagulation. Patients with irreversible risk factors or idiopathic VTE have a much higher risk of recurrence, as much as 26 % at 3 years [53], and these patients must have a risk/benefit analysis performed periodically to confirm the benefit of continued therapy. Guidelines recommend extended therapy beyond the initial 3 months of therapy for any second unprovoked VTE for patients with low or moderate bleeding risk [48]. Patients with a high bleeding risk should receive 3 months of anticoagulation. Patients with VTE and active cancer should receive extended anticoagulation over the initial 3 months of therapy regardless of bleeding risk [48].

Interestingly, heterozygosity for the factor V Leiden or prothrombin gene mutation does not substantially increase the risk for *recurrent* VTE [54]. Compared to an unselected group of patients with unprovoked DVT or PE, patients with circulating antiphospholipid antibodies probably have a higher risk for recurrent VTE [4]. The utility of other testing for inherited defects (e.g. measurement of protein C or S activity, homocysteine concentrations) in the assessment of VTE recurrence risk is controversial.

After a therapeutic course has been completed, a D-dimer assay can be performed, or a lower-extremity ultrasound with Doppler can be conducted, to assess for residual thrombus. A recent systematic review found an annualized risk of 8.9 % in those patients with a D-dimer > 500 ng/ml after a course of anti-coagulation (usually 3 months of warfarin) vs. 3.5 % in those with a D-dimer < 500 ng/ml [55]. A meta-analysis conducted by Douketis, et al. [56], in patients with a first unprovoked VTE who have their D-dimer level measured after stopping antico-agulation, found an annualized risk for recurrent VTE to be 3.7 per 100 patient-years in patients with a negative D-dimer result (either <500 ng/ml or <250 ng/ml depending on the initial study) and 8.8 per 100 patient-years in patients with a positive D-dimer assay (either >500 ng/ml or >250 ng/ml depending on the initial study). The hazard ratio was calculated to be 2.59 (CI, 1.90–3.32) for having an elevated versus a normal D-dimer result. The ability of the D-dimer assay to distinguish between patients with a higher and lower risk of recurrent VTE was not affected by the timing of D-dimer testing, patient age, or the assay cut point used (500 ng/ml versus 250 ng/ml) [56].

Treatment guided by lower extremity ultrasound with Doppler has been shown to reduce the risk of recurrent VTE by 36 % in adults with either unprovoked or secondary (provoked and reversible) first-time proximal DVT [57]. When the results were examined by subgroup (unprovoked and secondary), the findings were not statistically significant.

Ambiguity regarding treatment duration exists primarily in patients with unprovoked (i.e. idiopathic) DVT; therefore this should be the target study population. A prospective cohort study by Le Gal et al. [58] evaluated the risk of recurrent VTE in patients found to have residual vein obstruction (RVO) on compression ultrasonography of the proximal veins after completing 5–7 months of anticoagulation for unprovoked DVT. The researchers found no significant association between abnormal compression ultrasonography and risk of recurrent VTE (HR 1.4, $p = 0.19$) [58]. A systematic review published by Carrier et al [59] examining nine prospective cohort studies and five randomized controlled trials, concluded that the presence of RVO on compression ultrasonography was not associated with an increased risk of VTE in patients with unprovoked DVT (OR 1.24, CI 0.9–1.7). However, in patients with either unprovoked or provoked DVT there was a small increased risk of VTE in patients with RVO on compression ultrasonography (OR 1.5, CI 1.1–2.0) [59]. Studies differ in their protocols and many use two- or three-point ultrasound testing, which has lower sensitivity than whole leg ultrasound for diagnosing DVT.

Two clinical scores, DASH and HERDOO2, aid in the prediction of VTE recurrence [60, 61]. The DASH score uses the patient's D-dimer concentration, age, sex, and use of hormonal therapy to calculate a risk score that can aid in the decision to continue anticoagulation beyond 3 months [61]. The HERDOO2 score evaluates a number of risk factors for VTE in women and dichotomizes them into high-risk for VTE recurrence and low-risk [60]. High-risk women should continue anticoagulation beyond 5–7 months.

Post Thrombotic Syndrome

Post thrombotic syndrome (PTS) is a long-term complication of DVT. This syndrome occurs in 20–50 % of post-DVT patients (this includes mild PTS, severe PTS is much less common). PTS varies in severity, with the most common signs and symptoms being lower extremity swelling, pain, discomfort on ambulation, and pigment change. In severe cases, venous stasis ulcers may develop. Current guidelines suggest the use of compression stockings for prevention of PTS in patients with acute DVT [48]. Compression therapy should begin as soon as possible after initiating anticoagulation therapy and, when continued for at least 2 years after acute DVT in clinical trials, has reduced the occurrence of PTS by about 50 %. For the treatment of PTS, a trial of compression stockings is suggested [48].

New Agents

Dabigatran etexilate was studied in over 2,500 patients with acute DVT with or without PE (~20 % with PE) compared to standard warfarin therapy [62]. All patients received standard initial therapy for approximately 5–7 days with UFH or LMWH and were then randomized to dabigatran or warfarin. Dabigatran proved to be non-inferior to warfarin for the primary outcome of recurrent symptomatic VTE over the next

6 months and it resulted in a significant reduction in the combination of major and clinically relevant non-major bleeding (Table 5.16). Rivaroxaban has also been studied for the treatment of DVT, but in this trial, patients were randomized at the start of therapy to receive either rivaroxaban alone, or LMWH followed by warfarin [63]. Rivaroxaban was noninferior to the control arm for the recurrence of symptomatic VTE and resulted in a similar incidence of major or clinically relevant non-major bleeding over the course of followup [63] (Table 5.16). A recently published study examined the efficacy of rivaroxaban in the treatment of symptomatic PE, with or without DVT [64]. This study compared rivaroxaban alone (15mg twice daily for 3 weeks followed by 20mg daily for 3, 6, or 12 months) to enoxaparin followed by a VKA [64]. Rivaroxaban alone was noninferior to enoxaparin followed by a VKA in preventing symptomatic, recurrent VTE, with a decrease in major bleeding [64]. Apixaban is currently undergoing a phase 3 trial (AMPLIFY) for the treatment of acute DVT/PE and results are pending.

Stroke Prevention in Atrial Fibrillation

Epidemiology

Atrial fibrillation (AF) is a supraventricular tachyarrhythmia characterized by uncoordinated atrial activation [65]. AF is the most common sustained cardiac arrhythmia [66] and affects nearly 2.5 million people in the United States [67]. The prevalence of atrial fibrillation is directly related to age, with the frequency increasing after age 60 [67]. The average age of those with atrial fibrillation is 72 and this condition is more common in men than women [67].

Atrial fibrillation can be classified according to recurrence and persistence of the arrhythmia. A given patient will have a first documented episode; if the patient has another episode, the AF is termed *recurrent* AF [65]. If a patient has recurrent AF that terminates spontaneously, this is termed

TABLE 5.16 Comparison of trials evaluating dabigatran and rivaroxaban for treatment of VTE

Study	Drug, dose	Number, duration	Indication	Comparator	Primary outcome measure	Primary safety measure	Primary outcome results	Primary safety results
RE-COVER [62]	Dabigatran 150 mg BID, after 7 days of standard treatment	2,564, 6 months	Treatment of acute VTE	UFH or LMWH to Warfarin (INR 2–3)	Recurrent VTE and related deaths	Major bleeding	Dab: 2.4 %, 30/1, 274 Warf: 2.1 %, 27/1,265, HR: 1.10 (CI: 0.65–1.84) *Dabigatran noninferior*	Dab: 1.6 %, 20/1,274 Warf: 1.9 %, 24/1.265, HR: 0.82 (CI: 0.45–1.48) *No increase in major bleeding with dabigatran*
RE-COVER II [87]	Dabigatran 150 mg BID, after 5–11 days of LMWH or UFH	2,568, 6 months	Treatment of acute VTE	UFH or LMWH to Warfarin (INR 2–3)	Recurrent sympto-matic VTE and VTE-related deaths	Major bleeding events	Dab: 2.4 %, 30/1,279 Warf: 2.2 %, 28/1,289, HR: 1.08 (CI: 0.64–1.8) *Dabigatran noninferior*	Dab: 15/1,279 Warf: 22/1,289, HR: 0.69 (CI: 0.36–1.32) *No increase in major bleeding with dabigatran*

	Rivaroxaban		Treatment of acute DVT (without PE)	Enoxaparin to VKA (INR 2–3)	Recurrent VTE	Major bleeding or clinically relevant nonmajor bleeding		
EINSTEIN-DVT [63]	Rivaroxaban 15 mg BID (3 week), then 20 mg daily, *starting immediately*	3,449, 3, 6, or 12 months	Treatment of acute DVT (without PE)	Enoxaparin to VKA (INR 2–3)	Recurrent VTE	Major bleeding or clinically relevant nonmajor bleeding	Riv: 2.1 %, 36/1,731; Warf: 3 %, 51/1,718, HR: 0.68 (CI: 0.44–1.04); *Rivaroxaban noninferior*	Riv: 8.1 %,139/1,718; Warf: 8.1 %, 138/1,711, HR: 0.97 (CI: 0.76–1.22); *No increase in first major or clinically relevant nonmajor bleeding with rivaroxaban*
EINSTEIN-PE [64]	Rivaroxaban 15 mg BID (3 week), then 20 mg daily	4,832, 3, 6, or 12 months	Acute symptomatic PE, with or without DVT	Enoxaparin to VKA (INR 2–3)	Symptomatic recurrent VTE	Major or clinically relevant nonmajor bleeding	Riv: 2.1 %, 50/2,419; Warf: 1.8 %, 44/2,413, HR: 1.12 (CI: 0.75–1.68); *Rivaroxaban noninferior*	Riv: 10.3 %, 249/2,419; Warf: 11.4 %, 274/2,413, HR: 0.9 (CI: 0.76–1.07)

CI confidence interval, *Dab* dabigatran, *DVT* deep vein thrombosis, *Enox* enoxaparin, *HR* hazard ratio, *LMWH* low molecular weight heparin, *PE* pulmonary embolism, *Riv* rivaroxaban, *UFH* unfractionated heparin, *VKA* vitamin K antagonist, *VTE* venous thromboembolism, *Warf* warfarin

paroxysmal AF. If a patient has recurrent AF that is sustained beyond 7 days, then the AF is termed *persistent* AF. Long-standing AF may lead to *permanent* AF. The term *lone* AF applies to patients younger than 60 without cardiopulmonary disease (including hypertension), and often has a favorable prognosis.

Atrial fibrillation is important both acutely and chronically. Patients can present with hemodynamic instability from rapid atrial fibrillation, often when associated with other cardiac comorbidities. Morbidity and mortality also results from having a chronic tachyarrhythmia, which alone can cause morbidity, but also has been etiologically linked to ischemic stroke and congestive heart failure [68]. The risk of ischemic stroke is increased roughly fivefold by 'non-valvular' atrial fibrillation, and even more in patients with AF in the setting of significant valvular disease. Additionally, atrial fibrillation-related strokes result in higher mortality and greater disability than strokes of other etiologies [69].

Atrial fibrillation can result in ischemic stroke via cardiogenic embolism. A fibrillating left atrium causes stasis of blood which predisposes to clot formation. Clot formation usually occurs in the left atrial appendage [67]. Once an atrial thrombus has formed it can embolize to the cerebral circulation as well as to the systemic circulation. Because of this risk, all patients with moderate- to high-risk atrial fibrillation must be considered for anticoagulation. Anticoagulation carries with it inherent risks, therefore the risk of stroke must be weighed against the risk of anticoagulation.

Rate vs. Rhythm

Any patient presenting with atrial fibrillation must have the resultant tachycardia controlled. This can be achieved via blockade of atrio-ventricular node conduction or by converting the patient to sinus rhythm. Control of the ventricular rate is termed *rate-control* and conversion to normal sinus rhythm is termed *rhythm-control*. The decision to proceed with a rate-control or rhythm-control strategy is determined by many factors. In a patient presenting with new or recent-onset AF, the first parameter to be evaluated is the hemodynamic status of the patient. If the patient is unstable then the physician must proceed with urgent cardioversion. If stable, the patient should have pharmacologic rate-control with beta-blockade or calcium-channel blockade. At this point it is the clinician's decision as to whether the patient can continue on oral pharmacologic rate-control long-term or whether pharmacologic or electrical cardioversion will be pursued. A reasonable alternative to pharmacologic cardioversion has increasingly become radiofrequency ablation [65]. Multiple studies, including AFFIRM and RACE, have explored outcomes as related to rate versus rhythm control. Unfortunately, neither trial confirmed the hypothesis that a rhythm control strategy reduces the risk of either stroke or all-cause death. [65].

Stroke Risk Assessment

A well-validated risk assessment tool exists to evaluate the potential for stroke as a complication of atrial fibrillation [70]. This risk assessment tool, named, *CHADS2,* uses individual risk factors for ischemic stroke to calculate a score that corresponds to stroke risk. *CHADS2* is an acronym with each letter corresponding to a risk factor for stroke. The risk factors are: *C*ongestive heart failure, *H*ypertension, *A*ge (>75), *D*iabetes mellitus, and *S*troke or transient ischemic attack (TIA) (Table 5.17). The two at the end of the score represents the number of points assigned to patients with a prior ischemic stroke or TIA; all other factors are worth one point each [70]. The calculated score will then be used to guide anticoagulation based on the individual patient's stroke risk profile (see below).

Bleeding Risk Assessment

Several investigators have looked into bleeding risk with the goal of developing a bleeding risk index. Two notable and

TABLE 5.17 Stroke risk in patients with nonvalvular AF not treated with anticoagulation according to the CHADS2 index

CHADS2 risk criteria	Score	
Congestive heart failure	1	
Hypertension	1	
Age >75	1	
Diabetes mellitus	1	
Stroke or TIA (prior)	2	
CHADS2 score	Patients (N = 1,733)	Adjusted stroke rate (%/year)
0	120	1.9
1	463	2.8
2	523	4.0
3	337	5.9
4	220	8.5
5	65	12.5
6	5	18.2

(Adapted from Gage [70])

validated scores are the *HEMORR2HAGES* [71] and *HAS-BLED* [72] scores. These scores take multiple bleeding risk factors into consideration and estimate a yearly major bleeding rate. These scores can be used in conjunction with an ischemic stroke risk score, such as the *CHADS2* score, to weigh the risks and benefits of anticoagulation for a particular patient.

Antithrombotic Treatment

Antithrombotic treatment guidelines have been delineated by the ACCP as well as the American College of Cardiology (ACC), the American Heart Association (AHA), and the

European Society of Cardiology (ESC) [73–75]. The treatment of atrial fibrillation involves two pathways – controlling the underlying arrhythmia and providing treatment to prevent thrombus formation and embolic stroke. Guidelines for control of the underlying arrhythmia are beyond the scope of this text, but it is important to note that arrhythmia management affects antithrombotic management, thus some aspects of tachyarrhythmia management will be covered.

Current ACCP guidelines use the *CHADS2* score described above to guide antithrombotic management [75]. Patients with AF who have a *CHADS2* score of 2 or higher (high-risk) should receive oral anticoagulation [75]. Patients with AF who have a *CHADS2* score of 1 (intermediate risk) should also receive oral anticoagulation [75]. The suggested oral anticoagulant is dabigatran, at a dose of 150 mg BID, for both high- and intermediate-risk AF patients [75]. In patients who cannot take oral anticoagulation, the combination of aspirin and clopidogrel is recommended [75]. Patients with AF who have a *CHADS2* score of 0 (low-risk) should not receive antithrombotic therapy [75]. For low-risk patients who choose to take antithrombotic therapy, aspirin is suggested over oral anticoagulation [75]. Patients with paroxysmal atrial fibrillation and patients with atrial flutter should follow the above guidelines [75]. A rhythm control strategy (pharmacologic or catheter ablation) does not preclude the need for anticoagulation and these patients should follow the above approach [75].

Patients with AF for over 48 h (or unknown duration) for whom pharmacologic or electrical cardioversion is planned should receive anticoagulation with either a VKA, LMWH, or dabigatran for 3 weeks before elective cardioversion and this anticoagulant should be continued for at least 4 weeks after cardioversion to sinus rhythm, regardless of baseline risk [75]. Beyond 4 weeks, the patient should be anticoagulated based on their individualized risk profile [75]. Alternatively, patients can receive immediate anticoagulation with LMWH, IV UFH, or at least 5 days of VKA prior to cardioversion, and undergo transesophageal echocardiography (TEE) to evaluate for thrombus. If a thrombus is detected on TEE, cardioversion should be postponed and anticoagulation should be continued [75]. The patient should receive a repeat TEE prior to re-attempting cardioversion. Patients with AF known to be less than 48 h should receive immediate anticoagulation with LMWH or IV UFH and proceed to cardioversion (electrical or pharmacologic) [75]. These patients should also receive 4 weeks of anticoagulation after successful cardioversion, regardless of the patient's risk profile [75].

The ACC and AHA recently published a focused update of their 2006 guidelines with comments on dual antiplatelet therapy and the oral direct thrombin inhibitor, dabigatran [74]. Regarding dual antiplatelet therapy, the update suggests that the addition of clopidogrel to aspirin might be considered in patients with AF who are unsuitable for VKA therapy due to patient preference or lack of compliance [74]. Clinicians considering this strategy may wish to know that the ACTIVE-W trial (VKA vs. dual antiplatelet therapy) found that dual antiplatelet therapy was inferior at preventing stroke, without decreasing the risk of bleeding [76]. Evidence regarding the use of dabigatran was evaluated by the committee, but no recommendations were made because it was not yet FDA approved for this indication. [74].

Four major AF trials have recently been published assessing the efficacy and safety of the new oral anticoagulants for stroke prevention in patients with non-valvular atrial fibrillation. Certain patients were excluded from these studies, most notably, patients with severe renal dysfunction. At the time of this writing, two agents (dabigatran etexilate and rivaroxaban) have been FDA approved for stroke prevention in non-valvular atrial fibrillation. The Randomized Evaluation of Long-term anticoagulation therapY (RE-LY) trial assessed, in over 18,000 patients with non-valvular AF, the efficacy of either of two doses of dabigatran (110 and 150 mg BID) given in blinded fashion to reduce stroke or systemic embolism compared to open label warfarin with a target INR of two to three [77]. The efficacy of dabigatran, 110 mg BID was non-inferior to, but significantly safer than warfarin therapy. The efficacy of dabigatran, 150 mg BID, was superior to, but no less safe than warfarin therapy (Table 5.18). Of note, rates of intracranial hemorrhage were significantly reduced with both the 110 and 150 mg doses of dabigatran compared with warfarin, but risk of major gastrointestinal bleeding was increased with dabigatran at the 150 mg dose [77].

ROCKET-AF (Rivaroxaban once daily Oral direct factor Xa inhibition Compared with vitamin K antagonism for prevention of stroke and Embolism Trial in Atrial Fibrillation) was the pivotal trial showing that rivaroxaban was non-inferior to warfarin for the prevention of stroke and systemic embolism in patients with AF [78]. This double-blind study assessed over 14,000 patients with non-valvular AF who received rivaroxaban 20 mg once daily (or 15 mg once daily for Clcr 30–49 mL/min) or warfarin (goal INR 2–3). These patients comprised a higher risk population than in the RE-LY trial with a mean $CHADS_2$ score of approximately 3.5 (Table 5.18). Rivaroxaban was non-inferior to warfarin for the prevention of stroke and systemic embolism with overall bleeding being similar, but with decreased rates of intracranial hemorrhage compared to warfarin (Table 5.18). Of note, rivaroxaban had an increased risk of major gastrointestinal bleeding compared to warfarin [78].

ARISTOTLE randomized over 18,000 patients in a blinded fashion to apixaban 5 mg twice daily (2.5 mg twice daily in patients with two or more of the following criteria: age ≥80 years, body weight ≤60 kg or Scr of ≥1.5 mg/dL) or dose-adjusted warfarin (INR 2–3) (Table 5.18). Apixaban proved to be superior to warfarin in terms of preventing stroke or systemic embolism; the apixaban-treated patients also had significantly less major bleeding and better overall survival [79] (Table 5.18).

Finally, the AVERROES trial compared the efficacy and safety of apixaban with aspirin in patients who were deemed to be unsuitable for warfarin [80]. Apixaban, 5 mg BID, produced a significant reduction in stroke or systemic embolism compared to aspirin 81–324 mg once daily with no statistically significant increase in bleeding rates (Table 5.18). Although

TABLE 5.18 Comparison of the four major trials of dabigatran, rivaroxaban, and apixaban for stroke prevention in atrial fibrillation

Study	Drug, dose	Number, duration, CHADS	Indication	Comparator	Primary outcome measure	Primary safety measure	Primary outcome results	Primary safety results
RE-LY [77]	Dabigatran 110 mg or 150 mg BID	18,113, 2 years CHADS: 2	Prevention of stroke in nonvalvular atrial fibrillation	Warfarin, INR 2–3	Stroke and systemic embolism	Major bleeding	Dab (110 mg): 1.53 %/year RR: 0.91 (CI: 0.74–1.11) Dab (150 mg): 1.11 %/year, RR: 0.66 (CI: 0.53–0.82) Warf: 1.69 %/year *Dabigatran 110 mg noninferior* *Dabigatran 150 mg superior*	Dab (110 mg): 0.12 %/year p-value: 0.003 Dab (150 mg): 0.1 %/year p-value: 0.31 Warf: 0.38 %/year *Dabigatran 110 mg lower major bleeding and ICH* *Dabigatran 150 mg similar major bleeding and lower ICH*

Trial	Drug	Details	Indication	Comparator	Efficacy endpoint	Bleeding endpoint	Efficacy result	Bleeding result
ROCKET-AF [78]	Rivaroxaban 20 mg daily	14,264, 707 days, CHADS: 3.5	Prevention of stroke in nonvalvular atrial fibrillation	Warfarin INR 2–3	Stroke and systemic embolism	Major bleeding and clinically relevant nonmajor bleeding	Riv: 1.7 %/year Warf: 2.2 %/year, HR: 0.79 (CI: 0.66–0.96) *Rivaroxaban noninferior*	Riv: 14.9 %/year Warf: 14.5 %/year, HR: 1.03 (CI: 0.96–1.11) *Rivaroxaban similar major bleeding and lower ICH*
ARISTOTLE [79]	Apixaban 5 mg BID	15,000, 18 months, CHADS: 2	Prevention of stroke in nonvalvular atrial fibrillation	Warfarin, INR 2–3	Ischemic or hemorrhagic stroke and systemic embolism	Major Bleeding	Apix: 1.27 %/year Warf: 1.6 %/year, HR: 0.79 (CI: 0.66–0.95) *Apixaban superior*	Apix: 2.13 %/year Warf: 3.09 %/year, HR: 0.69 (CI: 0.6–0.8) *Apixaban lower major bleeding and ICH*
AVERROES [80]	Apixaban 5 mg BID	5,600, 18 months, CHADS: 2	Prevention of stroke in nonvalvular atrial fibrillation	Aspirin 81 to 324 mg/day	Stroke and systemic embolism	Major bleeding	Apix: 1.6 %/year ASA: 3.7 %/year, HR: 0.45 (CI: 0.32–0.62) *Apixaban superior*	Apix: 1.4 %/year ASA: 1.2 %/year, HR: 1.13 (CI: 0.74–1.75) *Apixaban similar major bleeding and ICH*

ASA aspirin, *CI* confidence interval, *Dab* dabigatran, *HR* Hazard ratio, *ICH* intracranial hemorrhage, *Riv* rivaroxaban, *RR* relative risk, *Warf* warfarin

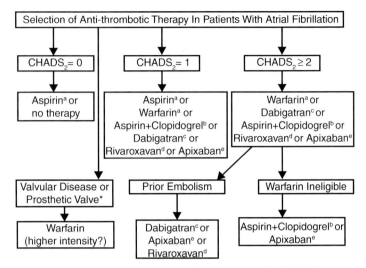

a: SPAF; **b**: ACTIVE-W, **c**: RE-LY **d**: ROCKET-AF, **e**: AVERROES and ARISTOTLE.
*mitral valve disease, a prosthetic heart valve, or mitral valve repair.

FIGURE 5.3 Selection and use of novel anticoagulants in patients with atrial fibrillation [81]

these efficacy results, compared to aspirin, are not unexpected, the AVERROES trial provides evidence that patients deemed to be at too great a risk for warfarin can be safely treated with apixaban.

The current ACCP guidelines [75] do not offer specific recommendations on the use of rivaroxaban or apixaban for stroke prevention in atrial fibrillation. Therefore, as these new agents become FDA approved for this indication, physicians must determine when it is appropriate to use each anticoagulant. To help guide physicians in this setting, a recent treatment algorithm (Fig. 5.3) has been published [81].

Prevention of Thromboembolism and Stroke in Patients with Valvular Disease

Prosthetic Valve Type and Location

Thromboembolic stroke risk in patients with prosthetic heart valves is evaluated according to valve type and valve location, since thrombus formation varies depending on these factors. Prosthetic valves can be divided into mechanical or bioprosthetic valves. Valve location is important because the flow of blood across the valve is directly related to risk of thromboembolism. Overall, the mitral valve is associated with a greater risk of thrombus formation than the aortic valve. This is due to the slower velocity of blood flow across the mitral valve, as well as an increased incidence of atrial fibrillation in patients with mitral valve disease [82].

Risk of Thromboembolism

The greatest risk of thromboembolism in native valvulopathy is in rheumatic mitral valve disease [83]. A patient with rheumatic mitral valve disease has a one in five chance of developing clinically detectable systemic embolism during the course of their disease [82]. This risk is increased further when combined with other cardiac pathology, such as atrial fibrillation. Early evidence showed an association between mitral valve prolapse (MVP) and stroke, but subsequent studies could not replicate this finding [83]. Therefore, it remains unclear whether MVP leads to an increased risk of stroke. Mitral annual calcification (MAC) also has conflicting evidence, and may cause an increased risk of stroke [83].

The greatest valvular stroke risk is associated with mechanical prosthetic valves. The location of the mechanical valve further determines the severity of stroke risk, with those in the mitral position conferring the greatest risk of stroke [83]. Bioprosthetic valves also confer an increased risk of thrombus formation, particularly in the first 3 months after valve replacement surgery [83]. Bioprosthetic valves in the mitral position are at increased risk of thrombus formation. As in the case for native valve disease, patients with prosthetic valves have an increased risk of stroke if they possess atrial fibrillation or other stroke risk factors.

Treatment and Outcomes

In 2012, the ACCP published guidelines on antithrombotic and thrombolytic therapy in patients with valvular and structural heart disease [83]. These guidelines detail when a patient should receive anticoagulation with a VKA (including the appropriate INR), when anti-platelet therapy is sufficient, and when no therapy is indicated. The new oral anticoagulants (e.g. dabigatran, rivaroxaban and apixaban), while effective for the prevention of stroke in patients with non-valvular AF, have not been studied in patients with prosthetic heart valves.

Anticoagulation in native valve disease is indicated only in certain disease states. Rheumatic mitral valve disease confers an increased risk of thromboembolism and when present with atrial fibrillation (AF), previous systemic embolism, or left atrial thrombus, anticoagulation with VKA (INR 2–3) is suggested [83]. Patients with rheumatic mitral valve disease and normal sinus rhythm (NSR) must have the size of the left atrium evaluated. For those with a left atrial diameter >55 mm, VKA therapy (INR 2–3) is recommended [83]. If the left atrial diameter is <55 mm, no antithrombotic therapy is indicated [83]. Although patients with MVP and MAC may have a small increased risk of stroke, there is not sufficient evidence to manage these patients differently from patients without these conditions [83]. There is no role for antithrombic therapy in patients with a calcified aortic valve [83].

Mechanical prosthetic valves always require anticoagulation with a VKA [83]. Immediately following surgery for the placement of a mechanical valve, the patient should be started on UFH (prophylactic dose) or LMWH (prophylactic or therapeutic dose) [83]. These patients will all receive VKA therapy, but the therapeutic target varies depending on valve location [83]. Patients with a mechanical valve in the *aortic* position should have a target INR of 2–3; if additional risk factors for stroke are present (e.g. atrial fibrillation), a higher INR target may be recommended [83]. Patients with a mechanical valve in the *mitral* position should have a target INR of 2.5–3.5 [83]. Double mechanical valve patients, and those with additional risk factors for VTE, should receive a VKA with a target INR of 2.5–3.5 [83]. All patients with a mechanical valve and low bleeding risk should receive low-dose aspirin in addition to VKA therapy [83].

Bioprosthetic valves also confer an increased risk of thromboembolism, particularly in the months after surgery. Current guidelines suggest that patients with an *aortic* bio-prosthetic valve receive low-dose aspirin for the first 3 months after surgery [83]. Patient who received a tran-scatheter *aortic* bioprosthetic valve should receive aspirin and clopidogrel for the first 3 months after surgery [83]. Patients who have a bioprosthetic valve in the *mitral* position should receive VKA therapy (INR 2–3) for the first 3 months following surgery [83]. After the initial 3 month period, all patients with bioprosthetic valves should receive long-term aspirin therapy [83].

References

1. Bagot CN, Arya R. Virchow and his triad: a question of attribution. Br J Haematol. 2008;134(2):180–90.
2. Khan S, Dickerman JD. Hereditary thrombophilia. Thromb J. 2006;4:15. doi:10.1186/1477-9560-4-15.
3. Baglin T, Luddington R, Brown K, Baglin C. Incidence of recurrent venous thromboembolism in relation to clinical and thrombophilic risk factors: prospective cohort study. Lancet. 2003;362:523–6.
4. Dalen JE. Should patients with venous thromboembolism be screened for thrombophilia? Am J Med. 2008;121:458–63.
5. Heit JA. The epidemiology of venous thromboembolism in the community. Arterioscler Thromb Vasc Biol. 2008;28:370–2.

6. Heit JA, Melton LJ, Lohse CM, et al. Incidence of venous thromboembolism in hospitalized patients vs community residents. Mayo Clin Proc. 2001;76:1102–10.
7. Cushman M. Epidemiology and risk factors for venous thrombosis. Semin Hematol. 2007;44(2):62–9.
8. Meignan M, Rosso J, Gauthier H, et al. Systematic lung scans reveal a high frequency of silent pulmonary embolism in patients with proximal deep venous thrombosis. Arch Intern Med. 2000; 160:159–64.
9. Ansell JE. Venous thrombosis. In: Creager MA, Dzau VJ, Loscalzo J, editors. Vascular medicine: a companion to Braunwald's heart disease. 1st ed. Philadelphia, PA: Elsevier Inc.; 2006. p. 743–64.
10. Leclerc JR. Natural history of venous thromboembolism. In: Leclerc JR, editor. Venous thromboembolic disorders. Philadelphia: Lea & Febiger; 1991. p. 166–75.
11. White RH. The epidemiology of venous thromboembolism. Circulation. 2003;107:I-4-I-8.
12. Falck-Ytter Y, Francis CW, Johanson NA, et al. Prevention of VTE in orthopedic surgery patients: antithrombotic therapy and prevention of thrombosis, 9th ed: American college of chest physicians evidence-based clinical practice guidelines. Chest. 2012;141:7S–47.
13. Gould MK, Garcia DA, Wren SM, et al. Prevention of VTE in nonorthopedic surgical patients: antithrombotic therapy and prevention of thrombosis, 9th ed: American college of chest physicians evidence-based clinical practice guidelines. Chest. 2012;141:e227S–77.
14. Kahn SR, Lim W, Dunn AS, et al. Prevention of VTE in nonsurgical patients: antithrombotic therapy and prevention of thrombosis, 9th ed: American college of chest physicians evidence-based clinical practice guidelines. Chest. 2012;141:e195S–226.
15. Caprini JA. Thrombosis risk assessment as a guide to quality patient care. Dis Mon. 2005;51:70–8.
16. Caprini JA, Arcelus JI, Hasty JH, Tamhane AC, Fabrega F. Clinical assessment of venous thromboembolic risk in surgical patients. Semin Thromb Hemost. 1991;17 suppl 3:304–12.
17. Rogers SO, Kilaru RK, Hosokawa P, et al. Multivariable predictors of postoperative venous thromboembolic events after general and vascular surgery: results from the patient safety in surgery study. J Am Coll Surg. 2007;204:1211–21.
18. Barbar S, Noventa F, Rossetto V, et al. A risk assessment model for the identification of hospitalized medical patients at risk for

venous thromboembolism: the Padua prediction score. J Thromb Haemost. 2010;8:2450–7.

19. Lederle FA, Zylla D, MacDonald R, Wilt TJ. Venous thromboembolism prophylaxis in hospitalized medical patients and those with stroke: a background review for an American college of physicians clinical practice guideline. Ann Intern Med. 2011;155: 602–15.

20. Qaseem A, Chou R, Humphrey LL, et al. Venous thromboembolism prophylaxis in hospitalized patients: a clinical practice guideline from the American college of physicians. Ann Intern Med. 2011;155:625–32.

21. Kakkar AK, Cimminiello C, Goldhaber SZ, et al. Low-molecular-weight heparin and mortality in acutely ill medical patients. N Engl J Med. 2011;365:2463–72.

22. Lansberg MG, O'Donnell MJ, Khatri P, et al. Antithrombotic and thrombolytic therapy for ischemic stroke: antithrombotic therapy and prevention of thrombosis, 9th ed: American college of chest physicians evidence-based clinical practice guidelines. Chest. 2012;141:e601S–36.

23. Eriksson BI, Dahl OE, Rosencher N, et al. Oral dabigatran etexilate vs. subcutaneous enoxaparin for the prevention of venous thromboembolism after total knee replacement: the RE-MODEL randomized trial. J Thromb Haemost. 2007; 5(11):2178–85.

24. Eriksson BI, Dahl OE, Rosencher N, et al. Dabigatran etexilate versus enoxaparin for prevention of venous thromboembolism after total hip replacement: a randomized, double-blind, non-inferiority trial. Lancet. 2007;370(9591):949–56.

25. Ginsberg JS, Davidson BL, Comp PC, et al. Oral thrombin inhibitor dabigatran etexilate vs North American enoxaparin regimen for prevention of venous thrombosis after knee arthroplasty surgery. J Arthroplasty. 2009;24(1):1–9.

26. Lassen MR, Gallus A, Raskob GE, et al. Apixaban versus enoxaparin for thromboprophylaxis after hip replacement. N Eng J Med. 2010;363:2487–98.

27. Lassen MR, Raskob GE, Gallus A, et al. Apixaban versus enoxaparin for thromboprophylaxis after knee replacement (ADVANCE-2): a randomized double-blind trial. Lancet. 2010; 375:807–15.

28. Lassen MR, Raskob GE, Gallus A, et al. Apixaban or enoxaparin for thromboprophylaxis after knee replacement. N Eng J Med. 2009;361:594–604.

29. Eriksson BI, Borris LC, Friedman RJ, et al. Rivaroxaban versus enoxaparin for thromboprophylaxis after hip arthroplasty. N Eng J Med. 2008;358:2765–75.
30. Lassen MR, Ageno W, Borris LC, et al. Rivaroxaban versus enoxaparin for thromboprophylaxis after total knee arthroplasty. N Eng J Med. 2008;358:2776–86.
31. Turpie AGG, Lassen MR, Davidson BL, Bauer KA, Gent M, Kwong LM, et al. Rivaroxaban versus enoxaparin for thromboprophylaxis after total knee arthroplasty (RECORD4): a randomised trial. Lancet. 2009;373(9676):1673–80.
32. Cohen A, Spiro T, Buller H, Haskell L, Hu D, Hull R, et al. Rivaroxaban compared with enoxaparin for the prevention of venous thromboembolism in acutely Ill medical patients. In: American College of Cardiology 60th Annual Scientific Session and Expo 5 April 2011; New Orleans, LA.
33. Goldhaber SZ, Leizorovicz A, Kakkar AK, Haas SK, Merli G, Knabb RM, et al. Apixaban versus enoxaparin for thromboprophylaxis in medically ill patients. N Engl J Med. 2011;365(23): 2167–77.
34. Glynn RJ, Danielson E, Fonseca FAH, et al. A randomized trial of rosuvastatin in the prevention of venous thromboembolism. N Eng J Med. 2009;360:1851–61.
35. Wells PS, Anderson DR, Bormanis J, et al. Value of assessment of pretest probability of deep-vein thrombosis in clinical management. Lancet. 1997;350:1795–8.
36. Wells PS, Anderson DR, Rodger M, et al. Evaluation of D-dimer in the diagnosis of suspected deep-vein thrombosis. N Engl J Med. 2003;349:1227–35.
37. Bounameaux H, de Moerloose P, Perrier A, et al. D-dimer testing in suspected venous thromboembolism: an update. QJM. 1997;90:437–42.
38. Frost SD, Brotman DJ, Michota FA. Rational use of D-dimer measurement to exclude acute venous thromboembolic disease. Mayo Clin Proc. 2003;78:1385–91.
39. Elliott CG, Lovelace TD, Brown LM, Adams D. Diagnosis: Imaging techniques. Clin Chest Med. 2010;31:641–57.
40. Bates SM, Jaeschke R, Stevens SM, et al. Diagnosis of DVT: antithrombotic therapy and prevention of thrombosis, 9th ed: American college of chest physicians evidence-based clinical practice guidelines. Chest. 2012;141:e351S–418.
41. Christopher Study Investigators Writing Group. Effectiveness of managing suspected pulmonary embolism using an algorithm

combining clinical probability, D-dimer testing, and computed tomography. JAMA. 2006;295:172–9.

42. Wells PS, Anderson DR, Rodger M, et al. Derivation of a simple clinical model to categorize patients probability of pulmonary embolism: increasing the models utility with the SimpliRED D-dimer. Thromb Haemost. 2000;83(3):416–20.

43. Wells PS, Anderson DR, Rodger M, et al. Excluding pulmonary embolism at the bedside without diagnostic imaging: management of patients with suspected pulmonary embolism presenting to the emergency department by using a simple clinical model and D-dimer. Ann Intern Med. 2001; 135:98–107.

44. Wicki J, Perneger TV, Junod AF, et al. Assessing clinical probability of pulmonary embolism in the emergency ward: a simple score. Arch Intern Med. 2001;161:92–7.

45. Sostman HD, Stein PD, Gottschalk A, Matta F, Hull R, Goodman L. Acute pulmonary embolism: Sensitivity and specificity of ventilation-perfusion scintigraphy in PIOPED II study. Radiology. 2008;246:941–6.

46. PIOPED Investigators. Value of the ventilation/perfusion scan in acute pulmonary embolism. Results of the prospective investigation of pulmonary embolism diagnosis (PIOPED). JAMA. 1990;263(20):2753–9.

47. Agnelli G, Becattini C. Acute pulmonary embolism. N Engl J Med. 2010;363:266–74.

48. Kearon C, Akl EA, Comerota AJ, et al. Antithrombotic therapy for VTE disease: antithrombotic therapy and prevention of thrombosis, 9th ed: American college of chest physicians evidence-based clinical practice guidelines. Chest. 2012;141(2 Suppl):e419S–94.

49. ATTRACT Study. Study overview and rationale. Washington University School of Medicine. 2009. http://www.attract.wustl.edu/dvt-study-overview.

50. Jaff MR, McMurtry MS, et al. Management of massive and submassive PE, ileofemoral DVT and chronic thromboembolic pulmonary hypertension: a scientific statement from the American heart association. Circulation. 2011;123:1788–830.

51. Aujesky D, Roy PM, et al. Outpatient versus inpatient treatment for patients with acute pulmonary embolism: an international, open-label, randomized, non-inferiority trial. Lancet. 2011;378:41–8.

52. Lee AY, Levine MN, Baker RI, et al. Low-molecular-weight heparin versus a coumarin for the prevention of recurrent

venous thromboembolism in patients with cancer. N Eng J Med. 2003;349:146–53.

53. Prandoni P, Noventa F, Ghirarduzzi A, et al. The risk of recurrent venous thromboembolism after discontinuing anticoagulation in patients with acute proximal deep vein thrombosis or pulmonary embolism. A prospective cohort study in 1,626 patients. Haematologica. 2007;92:199–205.

54. Goldhaber SZ. Deep venous thrombosis and pulmonary thromboembolism. In: Longo DL, Fauci AS, Kasper DL, Hauser SL, Jameson JL, Loscalzo J, editors. Harrison's Principles of internal medicine. 18th ed. New York, NY: McGraw-Hill; 2012. p. 2170–7.

55. Verhovsek M, Douketi JD, et al. Systematic review: D-dimer to predict recurrent disease after stopping anticoagulant therapy for unprovoked venous thromboembolism. Ann Intern Med. 2008;149:481–90.

56. Douketis J, Tosetto A, Marcucci M, et al. Patient-level meta-analysis: Effect of measurement timing, threshold, and patient age on ability of D-dimer testing to assess recurrence risk after unprovoked venous thromboembolism. Ann Intern Med. 2010;153:523–31.

57. Prandoni P, Prins MH, Lensing AWA, Ghirarduzzi A, Ageno W, Imberti D, et al. Residual thrombosis on ultrasonography to guide the duration of anticoagulation in patients with deep venous thrombosis: a randomized trial. Ann Intern Med. 2009;150: 577–85.

58. Le Gal G, Carrier M, Kovacs MJ, et al. Residual vein obstruction as a predictor f or recurrent thromboembolic events after a first unprovoked episode: data from the REVERSE cohort study. J Thromb Haemost. 2011;9:1126–32.

59. Carrier M, Rodger MA, Wells PS, Righini M, Le Gal G. Residual vein obstruction to predict the risk of recurrent venous thromboembolism in patients with deep vein thrombosis: a systematic review and meta-analysis. J Thromb Haemost. 2011;9:1119–25.

60. Rodger MA, Kahn SR, Wells PS, Anderson DA, Chagnon I, Le Gal G, et al. Identifying unprovoked thromboembolism patients at low risk for recurrence who can discontinue anticoagulant therapy. CMAJ. 2008;179(5):417–26.

61. Tosetto A, Iorio A, Marcucci M, Baglin T, Cushman M, Eichinger S, et al. Predicting disease recurrence in patients with previous unprovoked venous thromboembolism: a proposed prediction score (DASH). J Thromb Haemost. 2012;10:1019–25.

62. Schulman S, Kearon C, Kakkar AK, et al. Dabigatran versus warfarin in the treatment of acute venous thromboembolism. N Engl J Med. 2009;361:2342–52.
63. Einstein Investigators. Oral rivaroxaban for symptomatic venous thromboembolism. N Eng J Med. 2010;363:2499–510.
64. Einstein-PE Investigators. Oral rivaroxaban for the treatment of symptomatic pulmonary embolism. N Engl J Med. 2012; 366:1287–97.
65. Fuster V, Rydén LE, Cannom DS, Crijns HJ, Curtis AB, Ellenbogen KA, et al. ACC/AHA/ESC 2006 guidelines for the management of patients with atrial fibrillation—executive summary: a report of the American college of cardiology/American heart association task force and the European society of cardiology committee for practice guidelines (writing committee to revise the 2001 guidelines for the management of patients with atrial fibrillation). J Am Coll Cardiol. 2006;48:854–906.
66. Marchlinski F. The tachyarrhythmias. In: Longo DL, Fauci AS, Kasper DL, Hauser SL, Jameson JL, Loscalzo J, editors. Harrison's Principles of internal medicine. 18th ed. New York, NY: McGraw-Hill; 2012. p. 1878–900.
67. Singer DE, Albers GW, Dalen JE, et al. Antithrombotic therapy in atrial fibrillation. American college of chest physicians evidence-based clinical practice guidelines (8th edition). Chest. 2008;133:546S–92.
68. Conen D, Chae CU, Glynn RJ, et al. Risk of death and cardiovascular events in initially healthy women with new-onset atrial fibrillation. JAMA. 2011;305(20):2080–7.
69. Lin HJ, Wolf PA, Kelly-Hayes M, Beiser AS, Kase CS, Benjamin EJ, et al. Stroke severity in atrial fibrillation. The Framingham study. Stroke. 1996;27:1760–4.
70. Gage BF, Waterman AD, Shannon W, et al. Validation of clinical classification schemes for predicting stroke: results from the National Registry of Atrial Fibrillation. JAMA. 2001; 285(22):2864–70.
71. Gage BF, Yan Y, Milligan PE, Waterman AD, Culverhouse R, Rich MW, et al. Clinical classification schemes for predicting hemorrhage: results from the National Registry of Atrial Fibrillation (NRAF). Am Heart J. 2006;151:713–9.
72. Pisters R, Lane DA, Nieuwlaat R, de Vos CB, Crijns HJ, Lip GYH. A novel user-friendly score (HAS-BLED) to assess 1-year risk of major bleeding in patients with atrial fibrillation: the Euro heart survey. Chest. 2010;138(5):1093–100.

73. Camm AJ, Kirchhof P, Lip GYH, et al. Guidelines for the man-agement of atrial fibrillation: the task force for the management of atrial fibrillation of the European society of cardiology (ESC). Eur Heart J. 2010;31:2369–429.

74. Wann LS, Curtis AB, January CT, Ellenbogen KA, Lowe JE, Estes 3rd NAM, Page RL, Ezekowitz MD, Slotwiner DJ, Jackman WM, Stevenson WG, Tracy CM. Writing on behalf of the 2006 ACC/AHA/ESC guidelines for the management of patients with atrial fibrillation writing committee. 2011 ACCF/AHA/HRS focused update on the management of patients with atrial fibrillation (updating the 2006 guideline): a report of the American college of cardiology foundation/American heart association task force on practice guidelines. Circulation. 2011;123:104–23.

75. You JJ, Singer D, Howard PA, et al. Antithrombotic therapy for atrial fibrillation: antithrombotic therapy and prevention of thrombosis, 9th ed: American college of chest physicians evidence-based clinical practice guidelines. Chest. 2012;141:e531S–75.

76. ACTIVE Writing Group. Clopidogrel plus aspirin versus oral anticoagulation for atrial fibrillation in the atrial fibrillation clopidogrel trial with irbesartan for prevention of vascular events (ACTIVE W): a randomised controlled trial. Lancet. 2006;367:1903–12.

77. Connolly SJ, Ezekowitz MD, Yusuf S, et al. Dabigatran versus warfarin in patients with atrial fibrillation. N Engl J Med. 2009;361:1139–51.

78. Patel MR, Mahaffey KW, Garg J, Pan G, Singer DE, Hacke W, et al. Rivaroxaban versus warfarin in nonvalvular atrial fibrillation. N Eng J Med. 2011;365:883–91.

79. Granger CB, Alexander JH, McMurray JV, et al. Apixaban ver-sus warfarin in patients with atrial fibrillation. N Engl J Med. 2011;365:981–92.

80. Connolly SJ, Eikelboom J, Joyner C, Diener HC, Hart R, Golitsyn S, et al. Apixaban in patients with atrial fibrillation. N Eng J Med. 2011;364:806–17.

81. Viles-Gonzalez JF, Fuster V, Halperin JL. New anticoagulants for prevention of stroke in patients with atrial fibrillation. J Cardiovasc Electrophysiol. 2011;22:948–55.

82. Salem DN, O'Gara PT, Madias C, Pauker SG. Valvular and struc-tural heart disease. American college of chest physicians evidence-based clinical practice guidelines (8th edition). Chest. 2008; 133:593S–629.

83. Whitlock RP, Sun JC, Fremes SE, Rubens FD, Teoh KH. Antithrombotic and thrombolytic therapy for valvular disease: antithrombotic therapy and prevention of thrombosis, 9th ed: American college of chest physicians evidence-based clinical practice guidelines. Chest. 2012;141:e576S–600.

84. Bauer KA. The thrombophilias: well-defined risk factors with uncertain therapeutic implications. Ann Intern Med. 2001;135:367–73.

85. Eriksson BI, Dahl OE, Huo MH, et al. Oral dabigatran versus enoxaparin for thromboprophylaxis after primary total hip arthroplasty (RE-NOVATE II): a randomised, double-blind, non-inferiority trial. Thromb Haemost. 2011;105:721–9.

86. Kakkar AK, Brenner B, Dahl OE, et al. Extended duration rivaroxaban versus short-term enoxaparin for the prevention of venous thromboembolism after total hip arthroplasty: a double-blind, randomised controlled trial. Lancet. 2008;372:31–9.

87. Schulman S, Kakkar AK, Schellong SM, et al. A randomized trial of dabigatran versus warfarin in the treatment of acute venous thromboembolism (RE-COVER II). American Society of Hematology 2011 Annual Meeting; 12 Dec 2011; San Diego, CA. Abstract 205

88. Tapson VF. Acute pulmonary embolism. N Engl J Med. 2008; 358:1037–52.

Index

A. Ferro, D.A. Garcia (eds.), *Antiplatelet and Anticoagulation Therapy*, Current Cardiovascular Therapy,
DOI 10.1007/978-1-4471-4297-3,
© Springer-Verlag London 2013

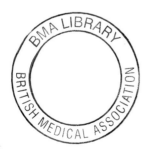

Printed by Printforce, the Netherlands